Prevention
LIFT LIGHT, GET LEAN

Prevention
LIFT LIGHT, GET LEAN

28-day weight-training plan for safe and easy weight loss

Brook Benten, M.Ed., ACSM-EP, and the editors of Prevention

CONTENTS

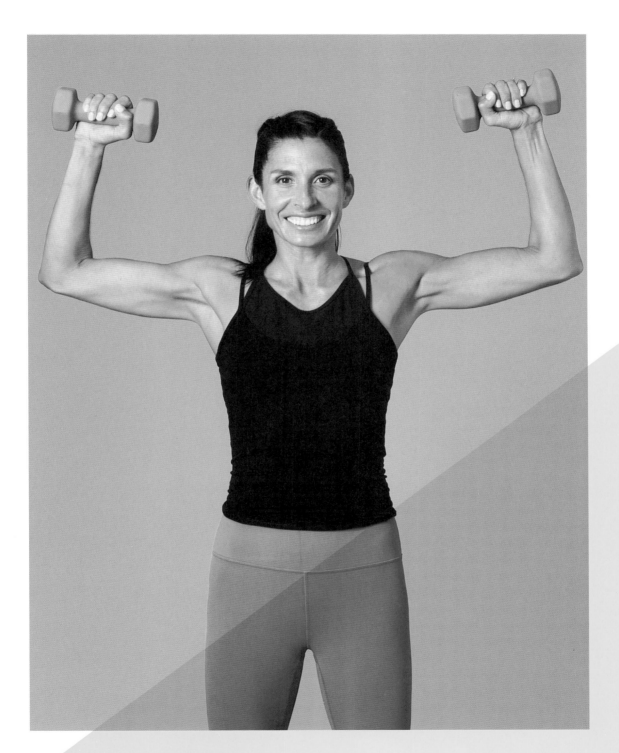

INTRODUCTION

Like many of the clients I've worked with in my 20 years as a personal trainer, I spent years as a cardio junkie. Running was my aerobic exercise of choice, and I believed that logging miles and miles each week—sometimes up to 50—was the most gratifying way to support my physical fitness and mental health. Until I got injured. (You saw that coming, right?)

My doctor diagnosed me with high hamstring tendonitis and gave me a stern warning: If I didn't take a break, the injury might not heal and could even get worse. With running off the table for a while, I needed to come up with new workouts that still got my heart rate up and worked my muscles. That's when I turned to light weight-lifting paired with low-impact cardiovascular exercise.

The plan I devised after my injury consisted of three days of light weight-lifting and three days of low-impact cardio like hiking with a weighted backpack, treadmill incline walks, and power walking interval workouts. It was gentler on my joints compared with running, but it changed my body for the better. I became stronger and more toned. And I kept up my cardiovascular fitness and maintained my lean body mass.

With a fitness approach as proven as weight-training, these results come as no surprise. I've seen a lot of workout trends come and go over the years, but the one that never goes out of style is weight-training. Whether you're lifting light, heavy, or something in-between, you're working wonders for your bone density, muscle tone, and body composition (percentage body fat).

If you're skeptical, I can understand that. It's easy to think that what worked for me may not work for you. The weight-loss industry is massive and it seems nearly every product promises incredible results. You should question any program that claims it will benefit your health in any way. As an exercise physiologist, certified by the American College of Sports Medicine, I give you solid advice that you can believe and take to heart. But light weight-training hasn't just worked for me, it's worked for women of all different ages and fitness levels. I've seen it in the data I've collected from conducting numerous research studies for *Prevention* on resistance training programs over the past decade. For example, in 2012 I led a study on a resistance training program that had participants use a 10-pound weight to perform 20 minutes of intense strength exercises (we're talking weighted burpees and all sorts of Satan-inspired cruelty, none of which will be found in the workouts in this book) three days a week, then walk three other days in the week. One average-sized woman in the study lost 13 pounds in merely six weeks.

As an inquisitive type who never stops thinking (anyone else feel like there are squirrels running amok up there?), I wondered if there was a better, kinder-on-the-joints way to treat the body that would achieve similar results. I wanted to try a low-impact resistance-training program using multi-muscle, multi-joint moves (with opportunities for participants to take breaks to refresh). This kind of program, I thought, would help people learn new mobility patterns and get their heart rate up, plus tone their muscles and lose weight if paired with low-impact cardio, nutrition, and smart wellness choices. Lastly, it would reduce nagging "owies" in key places, like knees, hips, lower back—now and later. So I built a program with 5- to

10-pound dumbbells and tested it on 20 women over two successive 28-day plans. The results were amazing. And now I'm sharing that plan with you.

Participants committed to the workouts in this book (Program 1 and Program 2), as well as to eating meals with non-starchy vegetables, consuming 72 fluid ounces of water a day and 25 grams of fiber per day, and doing intermittent fasting from 9 p.m. to 7 a.m. every day. They were also educated on the "3 Ss" for wellness (sleep, stress manage-ment, and social connections), which we'll get into on page 26. After 4 weeks on Program 1 and 4 weeks on Program 2, here's what we found!

The women who followed the plan reported impressive results. In just under two months, participants lost as much as 16 pounds and 14 inches—and you can do the same. These women were juggling real-life responsibilities—jobs, families, busy schedules. On top of it all, we asked them to begin this program right in the middle of back-to-school season! Turn the page to see a few of the incredible trans-formations and get ready to start your own.

Brook Benten, M.Ed., ACSM-EP

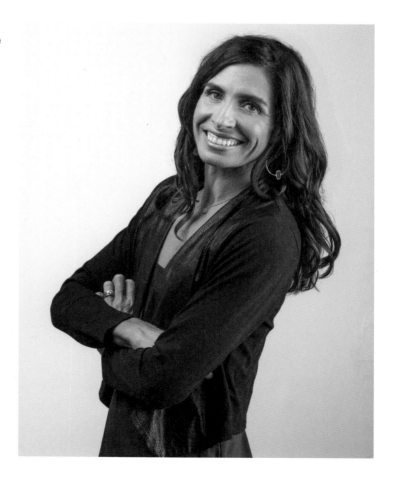

LIFT LIGHT IN REAL LIFE

By the end of the program, all 20 women in the Lift Light focus group lost weight and gained strength (and had fun in the process!). Check out a few of their stories here and get inspired.

STACY KELLEY

AGE: 51
POUNDS LOST: 8
INCHES LOST: 8.25

When Stacy Kelley completed the Lift Light, Get Lean program, she didn't just feel different from when she started two months prior. She felt different than she had in a long time. "After the eight weeks, I felt and looked better than I had in years," she says.

Despite having spent years doing different workouts, she says never tried anything quite like this mix of light weight-training and cardio. She noticed a change almost immediately, thanks to multitasking moves that help build strength and mobility, like sumo squats and Arnold presses. "After the first week, I felt a change in my muscles and flexibility," she says. "I hadn't done a workout like that before."

In addition to enjoying trying out the new exercises,

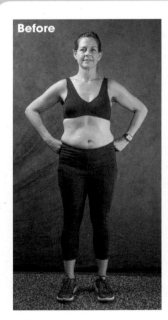
Before

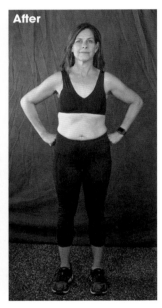
After

Stacy had no trouble finding time for the strength workouts, which take 20 minutes or less on average. To keep her motivation high and to stay accountable, she completed the program with a friend (because isn't working out way more fun with buddy?). Her efforts resulted in a loss of 8 pounds and a new fitness routine she says she would enjoy continuing to do regularly.

KELLY McELMURRY

AGE: 43
POUNDS LOST: 16
INCHES LOST: 14

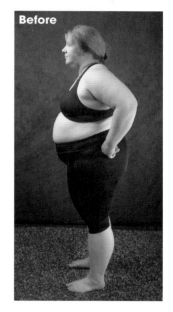
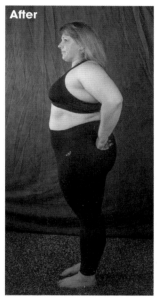

Like many people, when life threw Kelly McElmurry curveball after curveball, she found it difficult to maintain healthy habits. "There were many things happening in my life, the most significant being the passing of my dad," she says. "I had put my health on the back burner and let myself go."

Kelly says she often felt tired, got out of breath when walking, and could barely make it up a hill. She was in an unhealthy cycle and breaking out of it felt impossible. Lift Light, she says, was the thing that finally brought on change.

"I signed up, and that is when things started to turn around for me," she says. "Were the exercises challenging? Yes, but they were doable. I could do them at my own pace."

To follow the plan, Kelly only had to learn 18 highly effective exercises, which made sticking with it feel manageable. Each week she could feel her confidence growing while the numbers on the scale dropped. "Each time I accomplished something new, I'd get a little piece of my self-confidence back. I could literally feel myself getting healthier, and it felt so good!" she says.

In the end, Kelly lost an amazing 16 pounds and 14 inches overall—and gained a valuable shift in mindset that has helped break old patterns and get back on track. "Lift Light, Get Lean was my comeback, both physically and mentally," she says.

 Share your Lift Light, Get Lean progress with us on Instagram with the hashtag #liftlightgetlean and tag @preventionmag and @brookbenten.

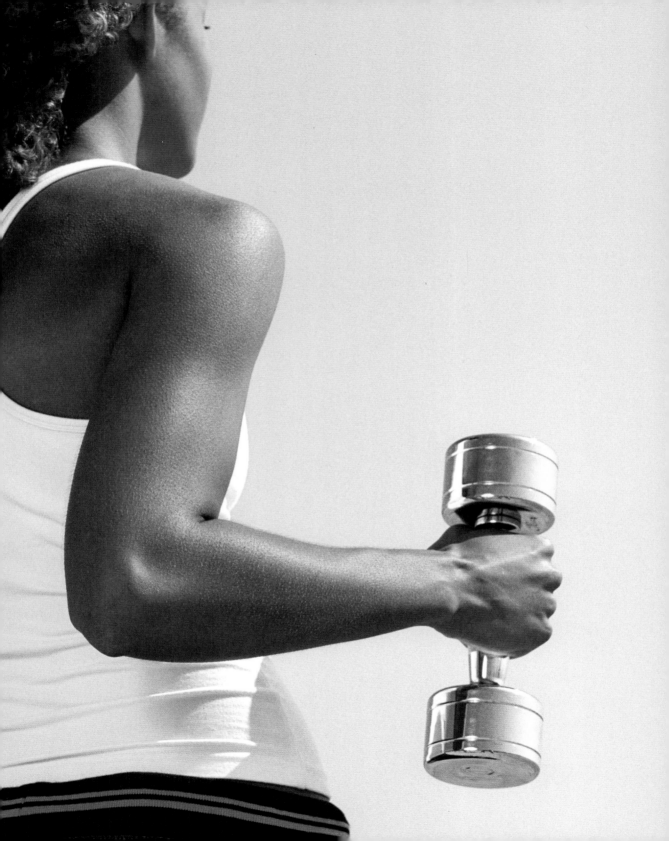

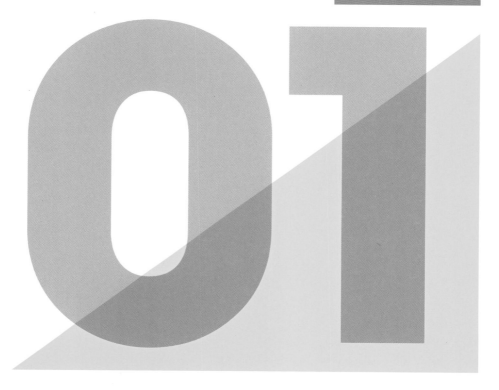

LIGHT WEIGHT-TRAINING 101

Maybe the traditional cardio plans you've tried before weren't enough to give you the leaner, more sculpted physique you were looking for. Perhaps you're on the hunt for a lower-impact workout routine that still manages to keep your heart rate up. Or maybe you're just starting to dip your toes into the exercise waters and want a simple, unfussy plan that will help you achieve real results. No matter what you might be seeking from your fitness routine, chances are that light weight-lifting combined with low-impact cardio, sound nutrition, and solid wellness habits can deliver.

What is light weight-training?

Light weight-training is a form of resistance training that involves lifting relatively lighter weights for several repetitions before taking a break. What one person considers a light weight may feel hefty to someone else, but as a general rule you should be able to complete more reps with a light weight (around 15 reps) than you can with a heavy weight (you may max out at 5 reps). In both of the 28-day programs in this book, you'll do a specific type of light weight-training, one that offers the most bang for your buck. These workouts include compound movement patterns, which recruit multiple muscles and joints simultaneously. For example, in a single exercise you might work your legs and shoulders, plus your glutes and core.

To top it off, these programs sneak in a burst of cardio. You'll perform a longer series of reps to really get your heart pumping before taking break. Talk about a double whammy.

Resistance training is any type of exercise that involves working your muscles against an opposing force. Think dumbbells, resistance bands, kettlebells, or even the weight of your own body. When performed regularly, it will support your efforts to preserve or build lean muscle tissue. It'll help make those muscles stronger too!

So what counts as "light?" The answer, as you might've guessed, depends on your individual fitness level. When performing a light weight-training exercise, the weight you use should be light enough that you can perform around 12 reps before your muscles become exhausted or nearly so. (That fatigue is a sign that your muscles are getting stronger!) But they shouldn't be so light that you finish a set feeling like you could still do a bunch more reps. Five to 8 pounds is the sweet spot for most women, but we'll talk about how to find the right weight for you on page 29.

The full-body benefits of lifting light

A light weight-lifting program can truly transform your body from head to toe. You'll become stronger and leaner, reap a slew of health benefits, and even get a mood boost. Let's take a closer look at what you can expect.

YOU CAN LOWER BODY FAT, LOSE WEIGHT, AND SCULPT A LEANER PHYSIQUE

It's no secret that aging slows down our metabolism and makes it easier to gain body fat, especially around the waist and hips. But regular light weight-lifting paired with regular cardiovascular exercise can make a difference. Combining the two builds lean muscle mass while burning calories, which can help you achieve a lower level of body fat. That's especially true when you pair resistance training with cardiovascular exercise, sound nutrition, and wise wellness choices. (I call these the Fab 4, and we'll talk more about them soon.) By the time you've completed this program, you might notice that your body looks leaner and more toned and that your clothes fit more comfortably.

YOU'LL PRESERVE AND BUILD LEAN MUSCLE MASS

No way around it: We all experience a natural decline in muscle mass as we get older. And less muscle mass means less strength. Over time, this can make it harder to do everyday activities that used to feel like a breeze—think carrying grocery bags or doing yard work.

The good news is that regular resistance training can help slow this decline. And holding on to more muscle mass means maintaining more strength. In fact, you might even build additional lifting capabilities. Either lighter or heavier weights will get the job done, but as we already mentioned, lifting lighter has the added benefit of boosting your endurance. In

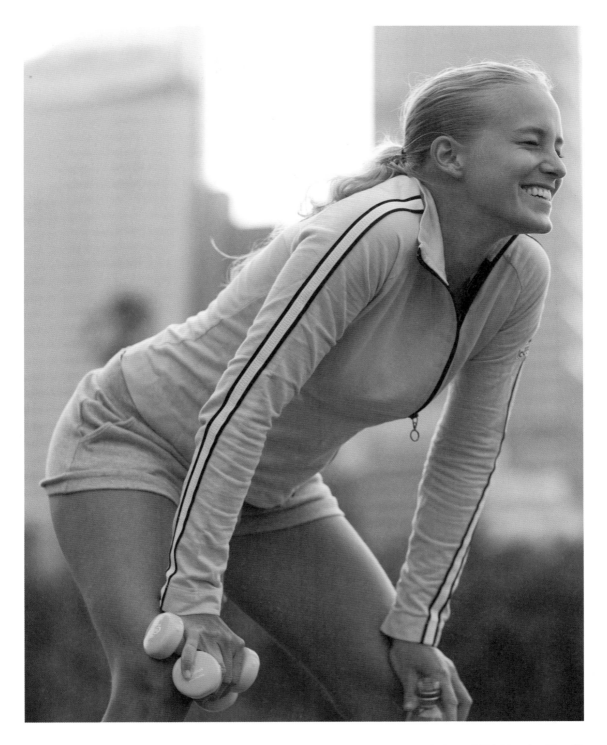

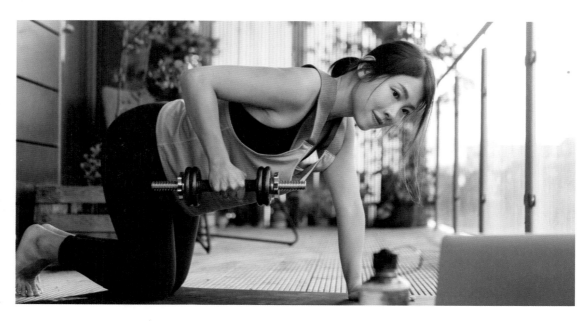

short, you're reducing the amount of age-related muscle loss, while keeping up your cardio fitness, too.

Just remember the importance of lifting the right amount of weight. In order to maintain muscle mass, you need to lift loads that challenge your current strength level. The body does a very good job of rising to the demands that you put on it. When you find that the equipment that felt light-but-challenging at the beginning of your program will start feeling very-light-and-not-challenging, it's time to make your muscles work harder by lifting a little more weight.

YOU CAN LOWER YOUR RISK OF INJURY AND ACHY JOINTS

Light lifting doesn't involve jumping, pounding, or sudden changes in direction, so there's less wear and tear on your joints. As a result, you won't find yourself sidelined by achy knees or ankles

after a workout. You're also at lower risk for getting injured while exercising, as long as you follow the instructions and perform the exercises correctly. And because it has fewer potential setbacks than workouts that pound your joints, light weight-training may also be easier to stick with in the long run.

YOU'LL BUILD A STRONGER CORE AND IMPROVE BALANCE

Light weight-training builds up the strength of your core, or mid-section, to give you a solid, steady foundation. I often say it feels like your abdominal and back muscles are going from a limp, wet noodle to a sturdy two-by-four.

But the benefits of increased core strength are no joke. Stable core muscles make it easier to maintain proper posture as you go about your day (no slouching!) and better protect your body when sudden movement changes happen. They also enable you to shift

or change directions quickly, like avoiding a crack in the sidewalk that could cause you to trip. And if you do start to fall, you'll be more likely to stabilize yourself and regain your footing quickly.

YOU CAN IMPROVE YOUR BONE DENSITY

Perimenopausal and post-menopausal women are at higher risk for osteoporosis, thanks to declining levels of bone-protecting hormones like estrogen and progesterone. But weight-training can help keep your bones sturdy and reduce your risk for fractures. The mild stress placed on bones during resistance exercise actually encourages cells to form new bone. This can offset age-related declines in bone health and even improve your bone mineral density.

YOU'LL SUPPORT YOUR HEART HEALTH

Walking, jogging, or bicycling might be the first things that come to mind when you think of exercising for your ticker. But aerobic activities aren't the only ones that do your heart good. Regular resistance training can significantly slash your risk for heart disease or a stroke. Greater muscle mass seems to make it easier for the body to maintain healthy blood sugar levels, which could help keep inflammation in check and ultimately protect your heart. Just a few weeks of weight-training can also help you lower your blood pressure.

YOU'LL REDUCE YOUR RISK OF DIABETES

We mentioned how muscle mass seems to make it easier for the body to maintain normal blood sugar levels. That, in turn, can help your body use insulin more efficiently and reduce the risk for developing type 2 diabetes. Regular resistance training can make it easier to manage existing diabetes and help reduce your risk for complications, too.

YOU'LL BOOST YOUR MOOD AND PROTECT YOUR BRAIN

Light weight-lifting isn't just good for your body. Exercise releases feel-good chemicals such as endorphins and serotonin and reduces levels of stress hormones like cortisol and adrenaline. Plus, there's no denying that satisfying sense of accomplishment that comes from finishing a tough workout. It's no wonder

that there's a strong correlation between higher physical activity levels and greater self-reported happiness, self-efficacy, and life satisfaction in older adults.

Regular strength training has also been tied to improved cognition in older adults. While experts are still learning about the relationship between resistance exercise and brain health, lifting weights seems to have a protective effect on areas of the brain related to learning and memory. In other words, stronger muscles just might keep your mind sharp.

The Best (and Worst) Ways to Use Light Weights

To see real results with light weight-training, you need a strategy. Follow these tips.

DO:
- Lift a challenging but manageable load for an extended period of time or more than 12 reps (for most women, that's approximately 8 pounds).
- Perform compound movement patterns, which recruit multiple muscles and joints.
- Focus on major muscle groups (glutes, quads, hamstrings, back, chest, shoulders, triceps, biceps, and core).
- Include movements in all three planes of motion: sagittal (forward and backward), frontal (lateral and side to side), and transverse (rotational).
- Stick to exercises that fatigue your muscles by the end of the set or circuit.
- Change your routine if you never experience some soreness post-workout. Delayed onset muscle soreness (DOMS) indicates microscopic tears in the muscles that enable them to grow stronger.

DON'T:
- Lift a load that's too easy.
- Perform only single-joint, stationary exercises (compound movements give more bang for your buck).
- Exclusively focus on small muscle groups (hands, calves, shins, and adductors).
- Limit movement to one plane.
- Spend time on exercises that don't fatigue your muscles by the end of the set or circuit.

Why does light weight-training work?

Resistance training improves strength and preserves or builds lean body mass by challenging your muscles. When your muscles are worked to the point where they're fatigued, the fibers develop tiny tears. (These translate to mild muscle soreness a day or so after your workout.) As the body repairs these tears, the muscles grow back stronger.

You don't need to start hoisting super-heavy weights to get these benefits. Heavy weight-lifting, which usually involves lifting the heaviest weight you can for 1 to 8 reps, can be a way to make muscles bigger depending on the amount of muscle-building

hormones present, known as androgens. Don't be afraid of lifting heavy, but it's not the only way to get stronger. Lifting lighter weights for greater reps won't give you massive biceps or quads, but it will help you achieve a toned look from head to toe. The higher rep count will also build your endurance and burn calories, so you'll improve your strength and, over time, lose excess body fat.

One important thing to remember: Light weight-lifting is only effective when you use a weight that's challenging enough to make your muscles very tired by the last rep, to the point where you could only eke out one or two more reps with clean form. That's the level of fatigue you need to hit in order for the muscles to get stronger and more toned.

Finally, you'll reap the biggest fitness benefits when you combine light weight-lifting with the other key pillars of healthy living: cardiovascular exercise, sound nutrition,

and wise wellness choices. These Fab 4 elements, as mentioned earlier, provide a quadruple threat that can help you build muscle and melt fat while nourishing your body and your mind. We'll talk more about the benefits of these principles and how to work them into your lifestyle on page 20.

What you need for light weight-training

The short answer is: not much! You might assume that in order to really work your muscles, a gym full of machines and equipment is a must. But in fact, all you need to complete this program—and get stronger and leaner—is a set of dumbbells. It's that simple.

Resistance bands, medicine balls, kettlebells, and barbells can all be great options. But dumbbells, with their extreme versatility, can replace all of those bells and whistles (pun intended). So when you need one piece of equipment that does it all, choose dumbbells. They make it easy to perform exercises with a little extra weight to effectively challenge every muscle in your body. They're also easy to hold and grip, so you don't have to worry about a weight flying out of your hand mid-exercise.

Dumbbells vs. Kettlebells

More than just appearance sets these two weights apart. One big distinction? The distribution of weight. The bulk of a kettlebell hangs below your hand when you grasp it, instead of level with it as with dumbbells. This means you need advanced core strength when swinging the kettlebell, because the fluctuating resistance can throw off your center of gravity. To learn complex kettlebell moves safely you can start by using dumbbells. The fact that the dumbbell's weight remains stable in your hand at all times makes dumbbells an excellent tool for learning the motions you can later apply with a kettlebell (if you wish).

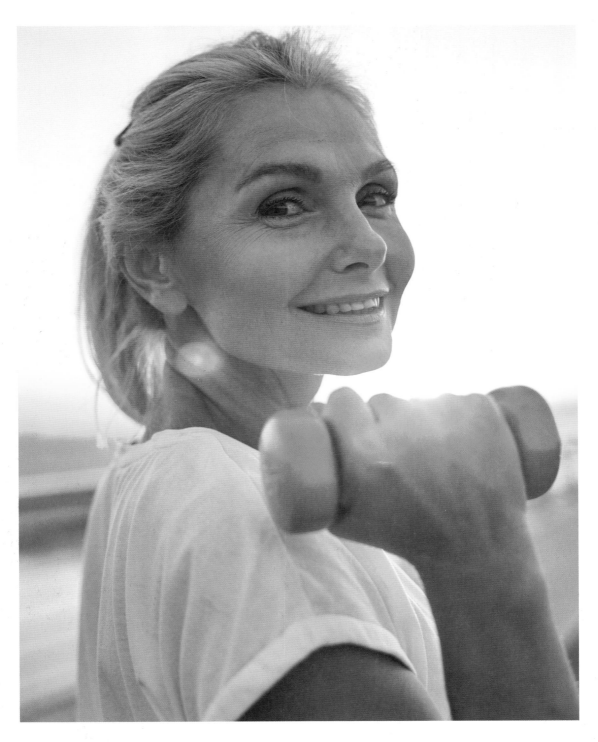

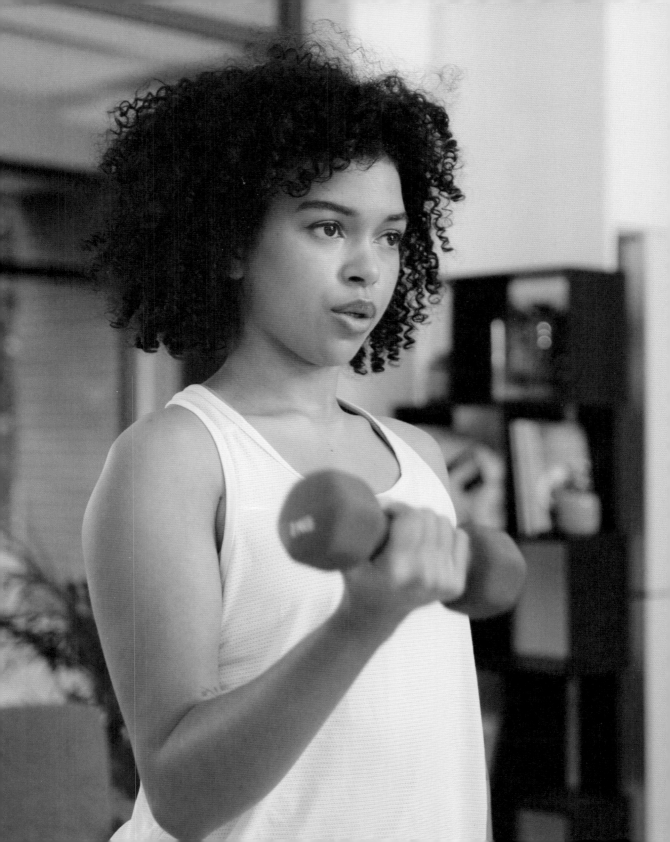

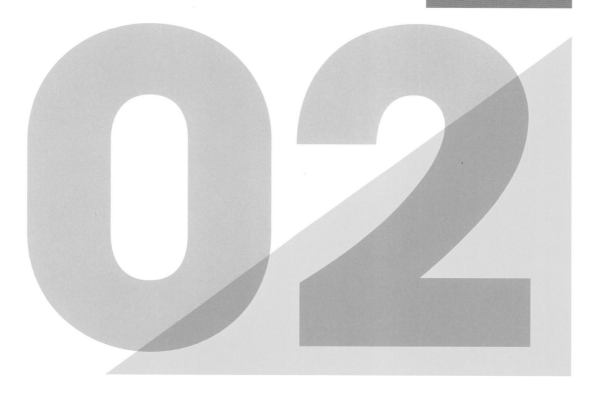

HOW TO GET REAL RESULTS

Just the fact that you bought this book means you're serious about getting stronger and leaner. To turn your fitness goals into reality, stick with these strategies.

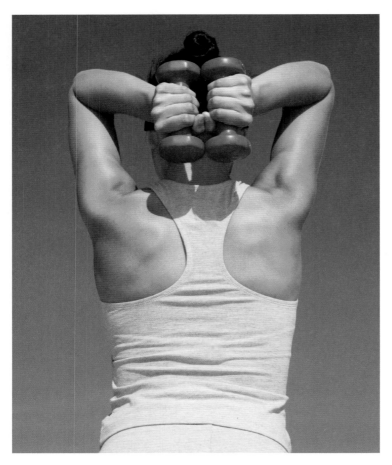

Follow the Fab 4

Light weight-lifting can change your body and improve your health. For some, just performing the resistance exercises in this program may be enough to get a little more toned and lose some body fat. But you'll get the best results when you pair light lifting with a few other key players. Together, I call them the Fab 4.

I mentioned the Fab 4 in passing a little earlier, and we've talked at length about the value of resistance training. Now, let's chat about the other three components.

CARDIOVASCULAR EXERCISE

Light weight-training by itself will do your body good. But it's the most beneficial when you pair it with regular aerobic exercise.

Aerobic exercises ramps up your heart rate and oxygen use, which improves your heart and lung fitness. When performed regularly, it can help you lower your risk for heart disease, achieve or maintain healthier blood pressure, and perform your daily activities without getting fatigued. Aerobic exercise also burns calories to support your efforts to lose fat and get leaner.

You'll do the most for your heart, lungs, and overall health by engaging in cardio exercise three days a week. It's a good idea

THE FAB 4

RESISTANCE TRAINING

CARDIOVASCULAR EXERCISE

SOUND NUTRITION

WISE WELLNESS CHOICES

to alternate weight-training days with cardio days to give your muscles a chance to rest. The cardio workouts in this program were designed to help you burn maximum calories to support your get-lean goals. (And all are low-impact, so they put minimal pressure on your joints.) But in general, any activity that gets your heart rate up counts as cardio. Think walking, jogging, bicycling, swimming, or going on the elliptical.

The resistance exercises in this program also deliver an extra dose of short cardio bursts to give you even more bang for your workout buck. Designed to bump up the intensity of your weight-lifting workout and raise your heart rate, the bursts raise your EPOC, or excess post-exercise oxygen consumption. And greater EPOC means more calories burned, both during your workout and afterward. You'll get a cardio burst from moves like front two-handed swings (p. 68), alternating swings (p. 104), high pulls (p. 74), and American swings (p. 108).

SOUND NUTRITION

Lifting weights alone may help you get stronger. But the path to a leaner, more sculpted physique also involves paying attention to your plate. Eating a wholesome diet can help you lose excess weight, and even more important, help you feel your best and protect your overall health. Plus, when you fuel up with the right foods, you'll have more energy

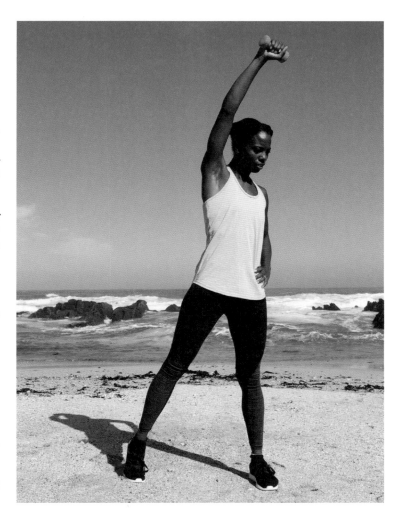

to give your all to every workout.

It's important to point out that there's no one-size-fits-all approach to eating well. Everyone has different nutritional needs, lifestyles, backgrounds, and traditions, and all of these factors are at play in figuring out what type of eating plan works best for you. That said, there are a few core nutrition principles that are always worth following. These are the universals that everyone should stick with.

MAKE WHOLE FOODS YOUR GO-TO

A diet rich in whole, minimally processed foods is best for reaching almost any health or fitness goal—including getting leaner. That means sticking with foods that you can easily recognize, and that haven't been altered much from their natural state—think an apple with peanut butter instead of a sugary apple-and-PB-flavored granola bar, or a baked potato instead of potato chips. The less packaging and the fewer ingredients, the better.

Whole foods deliver nutrient-rich fuel to help your body function at its best. Beyond contributing calories, the food we eat impacts everything from our hormones to our gut health to our metabolism. It also affects feelings of hunger and fullness, and may dictate whether you get hit with diet-derailing cravings. All of these factors can impact our ability to get lean and manage our overall health.

You might've heard this advice before. In fact, if you take a look at the different diets out there, almost all of them recommend choosing whole foods over their processed or packaged counterparts as much as possible. That's because when it comes to eating well, quality really does matter.

AIM FOR BALANCE AND VARIETY

Experts typically describe a balanced diet as one that delivers all of the nutrients you need for performance and healthy aging. But you can also think of it as a sustainable eating plan that makes room for everything—no cutting out foods or food groups. This approach will nourish your body and help you feel your best over the long haul.

The particulars of your plate may look different than someone else's. But in general, a balanced diet includes everything in the box to the right.

ELEMENTS OF A HEALTHY DIET

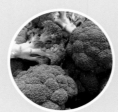

Vegetables: Eat a wide variety of different colored vegetables like broccoli, peppers, leafy greens, mushrooms, carrots, sweet potatoes, and tomatoes. Veggies get their bright hues from the nutrients they contain, so you'll consume the widest range of vitamins, minerals, and phytochemicals when you reach for the rainbow.

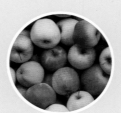

Fruits: Again, enjoy as many different types as you can. Choose whole fruit over fruit juice. A whole apple or orange, for instance, serves up fiber and other nutrients to help your body maintain steady blood sugar levels. But a glass of apple or orange juice has had that fiber removed, which can lead to big blood sugar spikes.

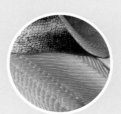

Lean protein: Pay more attention to the type of protein you eat and less to the number of grams you're getting. Lean protein sources like fish, poultry, beans, and nuts can help you preserve and build muscle tissue while lowering your risk for heart disease, cancer, and diabetes.

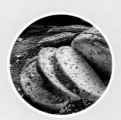

Whole grains: Reach for whole-wheat pasta, whole-wheat bread, brown rice, quinoa, or oatmeal over white pasta, white rice, or foods made with white flour like white bread, crackers, or cookies. Whole grains deliver more fiber to support steady, even blood sugar and help you stay satisfied longer. They also come naturally packaged with protein, fat, and other essential nutrients that support metabolism and energy production, immune function, bone health, and brain health, among other processes.

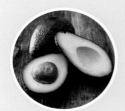

Healthy fats: Don't be afraid of fat! Just choose the good-for-you kinds most of the time. Poly- and monounsaturated fats—found in olive oil, avocado, nuts, and seeds—can protect your heart by supporting healthy cholesterol levels. Limit your intake of foods high in saturated fat like red meat, full-fat dairy, and baked goods. These foods may increase the risk for heart disease, especially when eaten as part of a diet rich in salt, sugar, and refined grains.

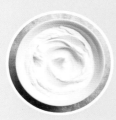

Low-fat dairy: Dairy is a controversial nutrition topic—some people recommend it as part of a healthy diet while others do not. One thing we know to be true is that some sources of dairy can be part of a balanced diet and other sources should be consumed less often. Plain yogurt and milk, for example, can deliver nutrients that support healthy aging, such as protein, vitamin D, and calcium. Flavored yogurts, ice cream, heavy cream, and processed cheese products, however, are vehicles for added sugars and saturated fat, so it's best to limit your consumption.

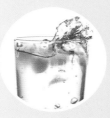

Water: Simple H_2O is your best bet for staying hydrated. (Unsweetened tea and coffee are okay too.) Juice, soda, sweetened tea, and sports drinks add extra calories without filling you up or providing extra nutrition. You may want to consider saving wine, beer, or cocktails for special occasions, too. Even moderate amounts of alcohol can make it harder to lose weight, especially around your waist, even if you exercise regularly.

You don't need to count food servings or measure out portions in order to eat a balanced diet. Instead, aim to fill half of your plate with vegetables and fruit, a quarter with whole grains, and another quarter with lean protein. Add healthy fats to your meals by cooking with olive or canola oil, for instance, or by adding an olive-oil-based dressing to your salad.

FOCUS ON THE RIGHT KIND OF CARBS

Many people think that they need to pile on the protein and cut their carbs very low in order to get lean. However, it's best to get a balance of calories from carbohydrates, protein, and fat. We generally recommend getting 45% to 65% of your calories from carbohydrates, 10% to 35% of your calories from protein, and 20% to 35% of your calories from fat.

Why are carbs helpful? Your body actually prefers to use carbs to fuel endurance exercises like the ones in this program, so a carb-rich meal or snack may help you push yourself a little further during your workout. Carbs are also a must for post-exercise recovery, helping you bounce back quicker.

Just pay attention to the types of carbs you're consuming. You'll reap the biggest benefits by sticking with complex carbs (like whole grains, beans and legumes, fruits, and vegetables) more often than simple carbs (like white bread, white pasta, candy, or baked goods). Complex carbs contain more fiber, vitamins, and minerals to support healthy aging, help maintain a healthy weight, and reduce the risk of developing diet-related diseases. They'll keep you fuller for longer, too.

DON'T FORGET ABOUT FIBER

Fiber is often overlooked and underestimated when it comes to healthy eating and weight loss. Incorporating fiber into your diet along with following the nutritional advice mentioned earlier can help your body function at its best and reach a healthy weight.

Fiber is a carbohydrate that the human body cannot digest. As it passes through the body undigested, it pushes waste and other toxins through and out the gut. Fiber also regulates the rate of food digestion and absorption through the gut, meaning it highly influences how, when, and which nutrients are absorbed. If food moves too quickly or too slowly through the gut, it can cause serious GI distress (e.g., nausea, bloating, distention, and pain), nutrient malabsorption, and could alter your gut bacteria for the worse. Adequate fiber consumption will also help maintain your blood sugar levels by preventing large spikes and subsequent drops. Plus, it's been shown to reduce the risk of developing various conditions, such as heart disease, diabetes, and metabolic syndrome (which may include high blood pressure, high insulin levels, excess weight, high triglycerides, and low levels of good HDL cholesterol).

The USDA's recommended daily amount of fiber for adults up to age 50 is 25 grams for women and 38 grams for men. Women and men older than 50 should have 21 and 30 daily grams, respectively. Choose foods that are naturally high in fiber, such as whole grains, nuts, legumes, fruits, and vegetables, rather than fiber supplements. Beyond fiber content, these foods are also nutrient dense, meaning they supply a lot of vitamins, minerals, and other beneficial nutrients that supplements do not.

EMBRACE THAT NUTRITION IS PERSONAL

There's no single dietary plan that works for everyone. Every body needs a different number of calories. Same goes for things like grams of carbs, protein, or fat. And we all have unique preferences: Some of us would rather graze throughout the day, while others feel better sticking with three square meals. Some of us like small sweet snacks each night after dinner, while others prefer to splurge on a bigger treat less often.

As for trendy diets? Some popular plans may help you lose weight, but if they don't mesh with your lifestyle you might have trouble sticking with them. If you'd like to follow a specific eating plan while on this program, we suggest intermittent fasting. Unlike other diets, which call for restricting your intake of certain vital macro-

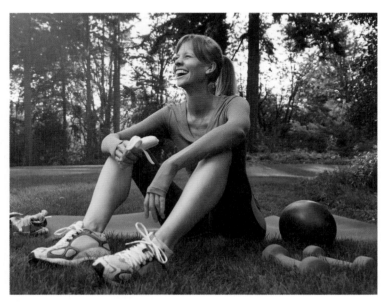

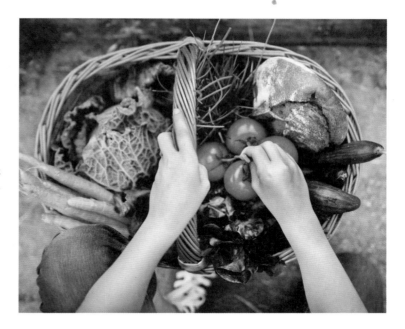

nutrients like fat or carbs, intermittent fasting focuses on when you eat. That means you can still incorporate the wholesome nutrition tips mentioned above and get the fuel you need to feel energized to take on every workout. Plus, many find it's easier to integrate into their daily life because there's only one directive you need to follow: Eat within a restricted time window every day.

For the 20 women who participated in the Lift Light Get Lean focus group, the eating window was from 7 a.m. to 9 p.m. In other words, they fasted for 10 hours each day, eating nothing past 9 p.m. each night and nothing before 7 a.m. each morning. Why those hours? Many people find that late-night noshing is their biggest nutritional struggle. So instead of tasking our group with remembering a bunch of "don'ts" (don't snack late, don't drink alcohol late, don't eat late heavy meals), we positively alleviated all of that with one simple "do": Fast from 9 p.m. to 7 a.m. As a result, all the women in our focus group were easily able to stick with the eating plan for the length of the program and shed pounds in the process.

Fasting helps promote weight loss by telling your body to burn fat instead of sugars. When you eat, you pump nutrients into your bloodstream that can be used for immediate energy and/or stored for later use, generally as glycogen and fat. In contrast,

when you fast, your body eventually exhausts the nutrients available in the bloodstream and is forced to start metabolizing its energy stores. When your body runs out of sugars available for use from the bloodstream or storage (i.e., glycogen), it turns to fat for energy instead. The process of moving from burning primarily sugars to fat is called metabolic switching.

Metabolic switching is thought to be the critical biological factor contributing to the touted health benefits of fasting. Such benefits include improved metabolic and cardiovascular health, blood sugar control, weight management, and improved cognition. However, much of the research showing biological benefits of intermittent fasting has been done with animals. The few studies done with humans conclude that intermittent fasting does not always promote greater weight loss or health benefits than typical

calorie restricting or consistent meal (e.g., three meals per day) diets. Moreover, when fasting you need to make sure you are not eating so few calories that your body starts to preserve energy stores (i.e., hold onto fat) because it thinks you're starving!

Intermittent fasting promises a lot. But it's not the right dietary pattern for everyone, especially those with diabetes or blood sugar problems. If you're interested in trying intermittent fasting, talk with your dietitian and doctor before starting to ensure you have the best personalized plan in place. Ultimately, we suggest starting simple with a focus on eating a variety of whole foods from each food group. You'll likely find that just eating a balanced, minimally processed diet will help you get leaner without making you feel deprived. And you'll be able to keep it up for the long term.

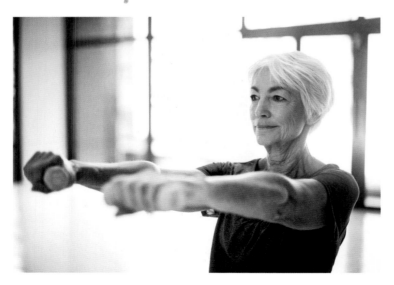

MANAGE YOUR STRESS

There's good stress, like the work that goes into planning a vacation, and bad stress, like finding a leak in your kitchen. A little bit of either can motivate you to get things done. But too much stress can become overwhelming: Instead of giving you an energy boost, you end up drained and unable to focus.

To keep your stress levels in check, you can:

- **Acknowledge your sources of stress.** When you take inventory of the tension, you can decide which situations are within your control and which aren't. Then you can make an action plan for managing the stressors that are controllable.

- **Keep your to-do list as short as possible.** If it's not a high-priority task, don't put it on your to-do list. Place it on a maybe-later list with the understanding that it might not get done.

- **Establish a simple meditation or mindfulness practice.** Time for reflection can help you maintain your perspective. But that doesn't mean you need to spend 15 minutes meditating every day. Taking five deep breaths when you first wake up or before you go to bed can do the trick.

WISE WELLNESS CHOICES

Regular exercise and healthy eating are musts for getting leaner. But health isn't just about what you eat and how much you move. You'll reap the biggest benefits from your light lifting program—and feel your absolute best—when you make the effort to get enough sleep, manage your stress, and nurture your social connections. Here's why these wellness targets—which I call the "3 Ss"—are so important, and how you can incorporate them into your routine.

GET ENOUGH SLEEP

The average adult needs between 7 and 9 hours of sleep per night. Logging enough shut-eye gives you the energy to power through your day, but that's not all. Adequate sleep is a must for helping your muscles rest and repair after exercising so you can give it your all for the next sweat session.

If getting enough snooze time is a struggle, these tips can help:

- **Establish a solid schedule.** A consistent bedtime and wake time will help get your body into a more predictable rhythm, so you fall asleep more easily.

- **Give yourself time to wind down at night.** Quiet activities like reading, meditating, or taking a bath give you a chance to relax so your mind isn't racing when you get into bed.

- **Pay attention to your environment.** A sleep-friendly bedroom is cool, dark, and quiet.

NURTURE YOUR SOCIAL CONNECTIONS

The people we surround ourselves with can influence our behaviors. Friends and family members who support your wellness efforts can encourage you to stick with your workout plan and other healthy habits (and help hold you accountable when your motivation starts to sag). To be at our best, we need other people!

Some advice for maximizing your social wellness:

- **Look for the like-minded.** We all have areas of our lives where we aren't able to choose who else is there—like at work, volunteer opportunities, or your kids' activities. In those situations, try to engage most with those who seem to share your wellness values and priorities. Notice a coworker who likes to walk outside during lunch, for instance? Ask if you can join them.

- **Ask for help.** Tell friends and family members about your wellness goals and ask them to support you in specific ways. Invite a friend to join you for workouts, or ask your partner if they'd like to establish a sleep routine with you.

- **Show your gratitude.** Express your appreciation to the people who are most important to you. You can literally say, "You are one of the most important people in my life, and I appreciate you so much." These kinds of verbal expressions boost well-being for both of you, research shows.

Be Consistent

You'll get the best results when you make the Fab 4 regular habits, which we'll help you do with the habit trackers throughout the 28-day programs. Doing a single light lifting session, having a salad for lunch, or going to bed on time one night are all good choices. And when good choices become your go-tos, you'll start to achieve real change. The queen of wellness is consistency!

That's not to say you need to be perfect. The key is prioritizing your time and energy according to what's most important to you, so healthy behaviors become the norm. Occasionally missing a workout isn't the end of the world when you know you'll get back to your regular lifting routine the next day. Treating yourself to pizza and ice cream for dinner is just fine when your usual menu is more wholesome.

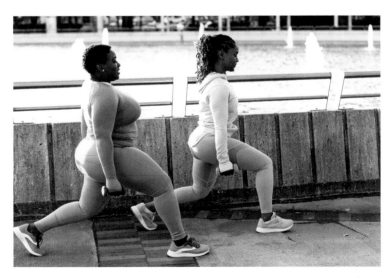

TIPS FOR
LIGHT WEIGHT-
LIFTING SUCCESS

Anyone can incorporate light weight-lifting into their fitness routine.
To make the most of your efforts, keep this advice in mind.

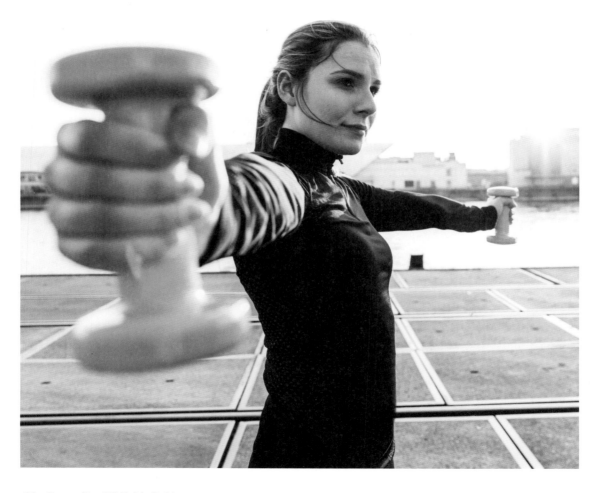

PICK THE RIGHT WEIGHT

Since you'll only be using one set of dumbbells for the entire program, it's important to choose your weight wisely. For the women in the Lift Light Get Lean focus group, that was somewhere in the 5- to 8-pound range. But your sweet spot may be lower or higher.

Your ideal weight should be heavy enough that it feels hard to get through the last few reps. At the end of a set, you should feel as if the set was challenging and uncomfortable, but doable. On the other hand, if you finish a set feeling like you could easily do several more reps, your weight is too light.

If you find that you're able to start this program using 10-pound weights, go for it. But if you need to start a little lighter, that's okay too. There's no glory in pushing yourself to the point of potential exhaustion or putting yourself at risk for injury. Listen to your body!

Finally, pay attention to when your weight starts to feel too easy. As your muscles adapt to the workouts and get stronger, you'll be able to lift more with less effort. You'll know it's time to bump it up to heavier dumbbells when you've reached the last few reps, but your muscles still aren't feeling taxed. Everyone can start strong, but if you're ending strong without some struggle, you're not giving your muscles enough resistance.

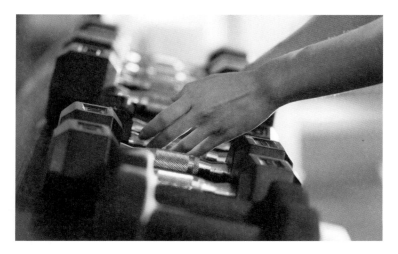

MAINTAIN YOUR TEMPO

Every weight-lifting rep involves two phases. There's the concentric phase, where you lift the weight and your muscle shortens. Then there's the eccentric phase, where you lower the weight and your muscle lengthens.

To help prevent injury, you should **exhale** in the concentric phase and **inhale** in the eccentric phase. Why? Pressure builds in your respiratory muscles when you inhale. Exhaling during the lifting phase will release that pressure, like a sigh of relief.

Let's use a biceps curl as an example: When you lift the dumbbells toward your shoulders, that's the concentric phase. You should exhale. When you begin to lower the dumbbells back down to starting position, that's the eccentric phase. You should inhale.

Lifting at a steady tempo involves matching your breath with these two phases while maintaining a steady pace. Given that a natural breath cycle is inhaling for two seconds and exhaling for two seconds, you can expect each rep to take four seconds. But there's

no need to bust out the stopwatch. Just follow the pace of your natural breath!

COMPLETE THE REPS THAT YOU CAN

Selecting a weight that challenges you and feels uncomfortable but doable takes trial and error. Your goal is to be able to complete each set, but sometimes you might not reach the finish line. And that's okay!

I encourage you to be bold and brave in your weight selection. After all, you won't know if a weight is the right fit for you until you try it. If a weight gets too heavy mid-set, though, stop using the dumbbells and finish the set using just your body weight. You'll still be lifting your limbs against the resistance of gravity, and that's something.

Ultimately, following through with the movements after dropping your weights is better than quitting on the spot or performing the entire program with too-light dumbbells. What doesn't challenge you won't change you. And you're in this for change!

Warm Up and Cool Down: It's Crucial!

Easing into exercise is always a smart move. A short warm-up raises your core body temperature and preps your muscles and tissues for more vigorous activity, which can reduce the risk for injury. And it doesn't have to be long or complicated. This simple circuit fits the warm-up bill for both resistance and cardio workouts, and it only takes six minutes.

Be sure to dedicate a few minutes to stretching post-workout as well. You can stick with some of the same moves you used during your warmup. Perform the hip hulas, lateral lunges with rotation, and hacky sacks for one minute each. (You can also try them on days when you've been sitting for extended periods of time!)

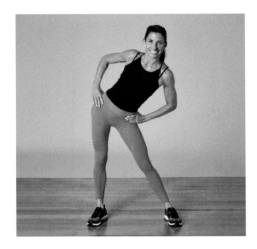

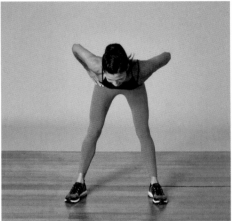

HIP HULAS

For hip mobility

HOW TO DO IT

SETUP Stand tall with your feet wider than hip-width apart and put your hands on your hips.

STEP 1 Rotate your hips in a clockwise circle. Keep your back flat, like the top of a table, when you push your hips back, and hyperextend your hips, stretching the hip flexors, when your hips circle to the front.

STEP 2 Rotate your hips in a counterclockwise circle.

TIME 30 seconds clockwise and 30 seconds counterclockwise

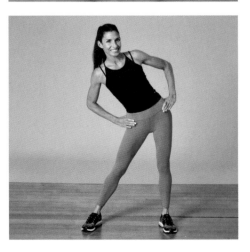

FRANKENSTEINS

For hamstrings stretch

HOW TO DO IT

SETUP Stand tall with your arms extended in front of you.

STEP 1 Kick your right leg up as close as possible to your right hand, then return to standing.

STEP 2 Kick your left leg up as close as possible to your left hand, then return to standing.

TIME 1 minute total

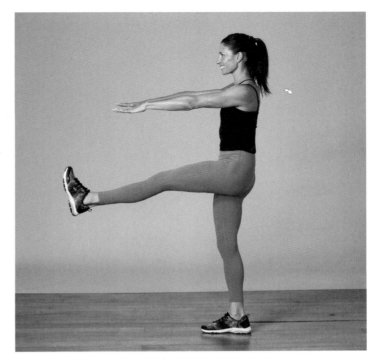

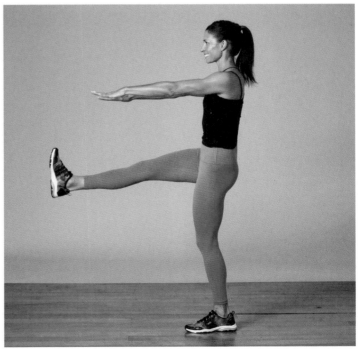

SHOULDER CORKSCREWS

For shoulder mobility

HOW TO DO IT

SETUP Stand tall with your arms extended out at shoulder height, forming a "T."

STEP 1 Shift your torso to the right and turn your right hand so the palm faces up. Hold momentarily.

STEP 2 Shift your torso to the left and turn your left hand so the palm faces up. Hold momentarily.

TIME 1 minute total

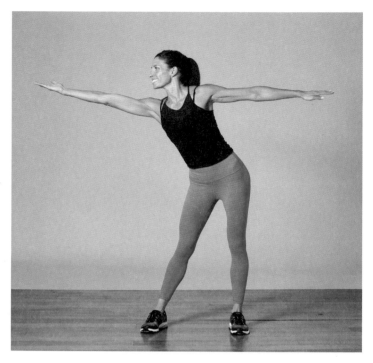

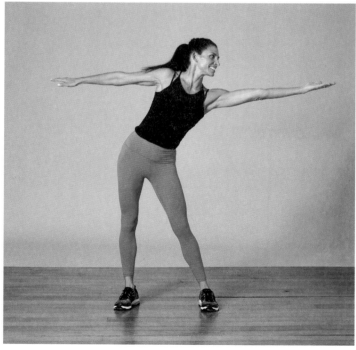

LATERAL LUNGES WITH ROTATION

For hip mobility, glutes stretch, chest stretch, shoulder mobility, and spinal twist

HOW TO DO IT

SETUP Stand tall with your arms by your sides.

STEP 1 Step your right foot out to the side. Touch your left hand outside of your right foot, and reach your right hand high to the ceiling. Look up toward your right hand. Hold momentarily, then return to the starting position.

STEP 2 Step your left foot out to the side. Touch your right hand outside of your left foot, and reach your left hand to the ceiling. Look up toward your left hand. Hold momentarily. Continue to alternate sides.

TIME 1 minute total

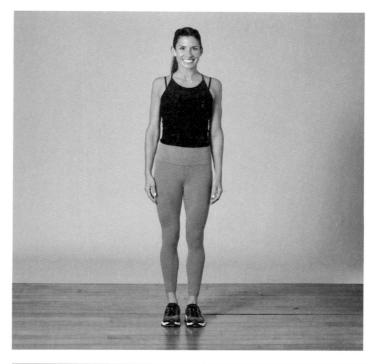

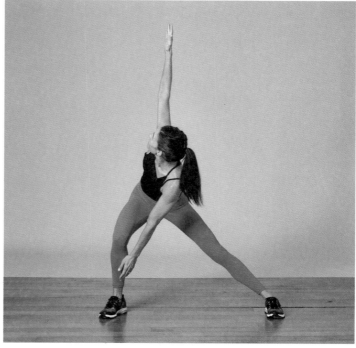

HACKY SACKS

For glutes stretch

HOW TO DO IT

SETUP Stand tall with your feet hip-width apart and hands by your sides.

STEP 1 Lift your left foot toward your right hand, touching your hand to your inner ankle.

STEP 2 Lift your right foot toward your left hand, touching your hand to your inner ankle. Continue to alternate sides.

TIME 1 minute total

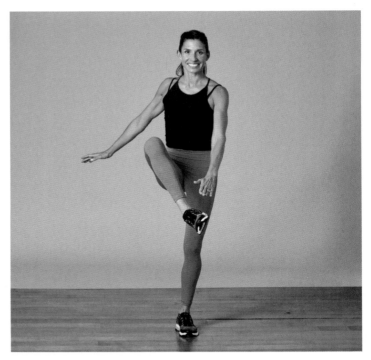

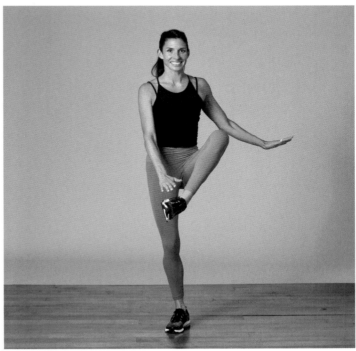

SUMO SQUATS TO STANDING ROTATION

For knee and hip mobility and spinal twist

HOW TO DO IT

SETUP Stand tall with your feet wider than hip-width apart and toes turned to 2 o'clock and 10 o'clock. Allow your arms to dangle from your shoulders.

STEP 1 Track your knees over your toes and lower into a plié squat, dropping your fingertips to (or nearly to) the floor.

STEP 2 Squeeze your glutes and rise up to starting position. Rotate your torso in one direction.

Repeat, rotating to the other side.

TIME 1 minute total

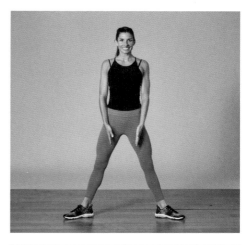

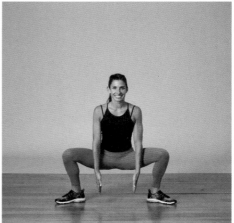

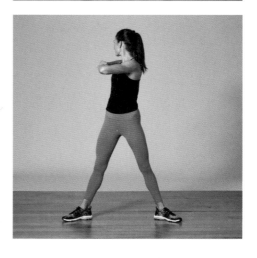

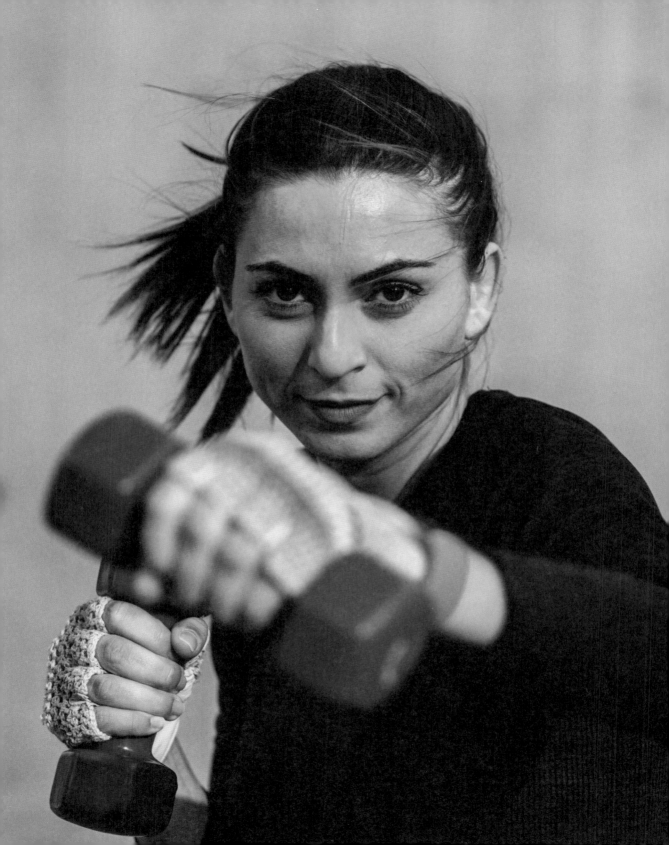

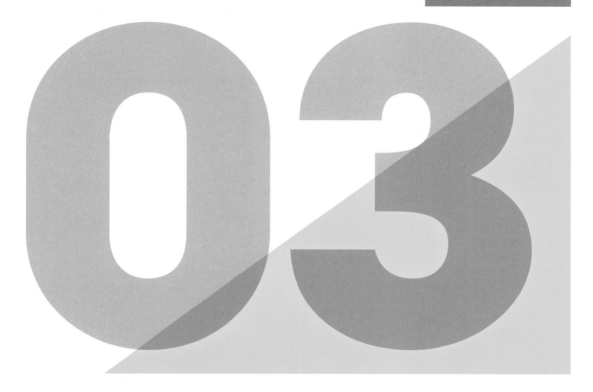

HOW THE 28-DAY PLAN WORKS

This 28-day, four-week plan utilizes light weight-lifting and cardiovascular work-outs to help you build strength, burn fat, and improve your endurance. Each week alternates three days of resistance training workouts with three days of aerobic endurance workouts, plus a day of rest.

Follow the plan while making wise nutrition and wellness choices, and you can expect to see the numbers on the scale start to drop by the end. Just as important, you'll have taken charge of your time, your choices, and your routine. After 28 days you'll have built a foundation of solid exercise, eating, and wellness habits that can support your health for life.

Pick your program

This plan has two programs designed to challenge people with different fitness levels. Both programs will test your endurance, core strength, and balance. The one you pick depends on your current fitness level and experience with weight lifting.

PROGRAM 1

This plan is for all fitness levels. It features multi-muscle and multi-joint exercises with moderately paced progressions designed for anyone with an injury-free, able body.

PROGRAM 2

Start here if your fitness level is intermediate or advanced or if you regularly do resistance exercises two to three times per week. The moves require some established strength—especially core strength—to perform properly. The progressions are low impact but high intensity.

Key Body Positions

Many of the exercises in this program rely on a few foundational positions. Here are some you'll see referenced throughout the workouts.

CURL: Arm position in which you bend your elbow and draw a dumbbell toward your shoulder.

HIP HINGE: Bent-over position in which you push your butt back, as if drawing your glutes toward the back wall. Keep your back flat (your back won't be vertical, but it will be flat).

LUNGE: Feet positioned so one is in front of you and one is behind you; knees are bent with front knee directly over front ankle and back shin is parallel to the floor.

QUADRUPED: Also known as "on all fours"; your knees and hands are on the floor with your wrists underneath your shoulders and your knees underneath your hips.

RACK: Holding dumbbells level with your collarbones, elbows bent.

SQUAT: Lower-body position in which your knees are bent and your butt drops down toward the ground while keeping your knees and toes tracking the same direction, whether that's straight forward or turned out to 10 o'clock and 2 o'clock.

	PROGRAM 1	PROGRAM 2
INTENSITY	✓	✓ ✓
CORE ENGAGEMENT	✓	✓ ✓ ✓
BALANCE CHALLENGE	✓ ✓	✓ ✓ ✓

LIGHT LIFTING WORKOUTS

These are the resistance exercises you'll do on Mondays, Wednesdays, and Fridays.

MONDAYS: LOWER BODY

PROGRAM 1	PROGRAM 2
• Front Two-Handed Swings • Forward Lunges • Curtsy Lunges • Lateral Lunges • Back Lunges • Sumo Squats	*Uses a Single Dumbbell* • Alternating Swings • Right Lunge Back with Dumbbell Swing Backs • Right Skater to Balance Holds • Rainbow Lunges • Left Lunge Back with Dumbbell Swing Backs • Left Skater to Balance Holds

WEDNESDAYS: UPPER BODY

PROGRAM 1	PROGRAM 2
• High Pulls • Pec Deck to Overhead Presses • Reverse Flys • Alternating MAC Raises • Supinated Rows (a.k.a., Biceps Rows) • Triceps Kickbacks	• American Swings • ISO Biceps Hold at 90 Degrees with Alternating Lunge Backs • Overhead Triceps Extensions • Reciprocal Bent Over Rows (a.k.a., Milk the Cow) • Arnold Presses • 90-Degree Lateral Raises

FRIDAYS: FULL BODY + CORE

PROGRAM 1	PROGRAM 2
• Squat to Presses • Right Leg Lunge Back to Biceps Curls • Left Leg Lunge Back to Overhead Triceps Extensions • Dead Lift to Scaptions • Sumo Squat to Upright Rows • Hip Abduction to Lateral Shoulder Raises	*These are tough, so consider starting with lighter dumbbells or using body weight alone.* • Traveling Bear Planks • Alternating Renegade Rows • Bird Dogs • Plank to Half Pigeons (alternating) • Hip Bridge to Crab Rotations • Flutter Kicks with Arms over Shoulders

You'll find full instructions starting on page 49.

Build your strength over time

Regardless of which program you choose, your light lifting workouts will get progressively longer and more challenging each week. That's a good thing, since each week you'll be stronger and able to work harder. Here's a quick overview of what to expect.

- **Week 1—Sets and Reps:** You'll kick things off with two sets of 16 repetitions to build muscular endurance. Rest for as long as you need between each set.

- **Week 2—Circuits:** By now, you've gotten a handle on how to perform all of the moves in the program. You'll crank up the volume by performing circuit-style rounds, only stopping to rest at the end of each circuit. (We recommend a two-minute rest, but you can take more time if you need it.)

- **Week 3—EMOM (Every Minute on the Minute):** In week 3, you'll perform two repetitions of every exercise, every minute starting at the top of the minute. (For any exercise that features alternating limbs, count the move on the right and on the left as one total rep, not two.) When you finish, rest for the remainder of the minute before moving on.

- **Week 4—AMRAP (As Many Rounds as Possible):** In the final week, you'll do the greatest volume of work over the longest period of time. You'll perform four repetitions of every exercise, resting for just 10 seconds before doing it all over again. When 20 minutes have passed, you're done!

Workout Words to Know

REP: Short for "repetition." One complete execution of an exercise. If the workout calls for 5 reps of a move, perform that move 5 times.

SET: One complete group of reps to be performed consecutively before resting. If the workout calls for 2 sets of 5 reps, perform that move 5 times, rest, then complete a second round of 5 reps.

CIRCUIT: A series of exercises to be performed one after the other for an extended duration before taking a break. If the workout is a circuit, perform 2 sets of all the moves one time. Then rest. Return to the first move and complete your second circuit of the exercises.

Alternate between resistance and cardio

Each week alternates resistance training days with cardiovascular days. Performing resistance exercises on nonconsecutive days gives your muscles a chance to rest and repair, allowing them to get stronger.

The plan is designed to primarily work different parts of your body on different days of the week, optimizing your time and turning up the dial on your metabolism. Here's how it breaks down:

- **Mondays:** Resistance training, primarily lower body

- **Tuesdays:** Cardiovascular endurance

- **Wednesdays:** Resistance training, primarily upper body

- **Thursdays:** Cardiovascular endurance

- **Fridays:** Resistance training, full body and core

- **Saturdays:** Cardiovascular endurance

- **Sundays:** Rest

It's important to have one day of rest each week so that your body can fully recharge itself. If you'd prefer to pick a day other than Sunday to rest, that's fine. You can shift days to make them work for your schedule. Just make sure you're alternating three resistance training days with three cardio days each week.

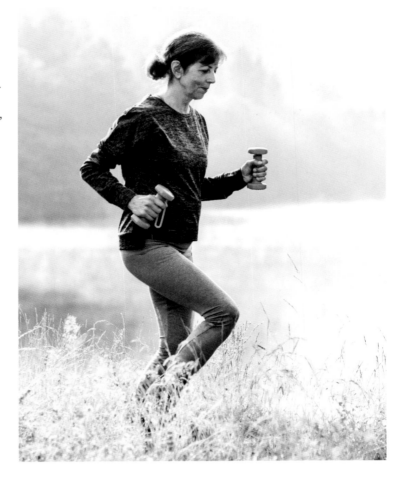

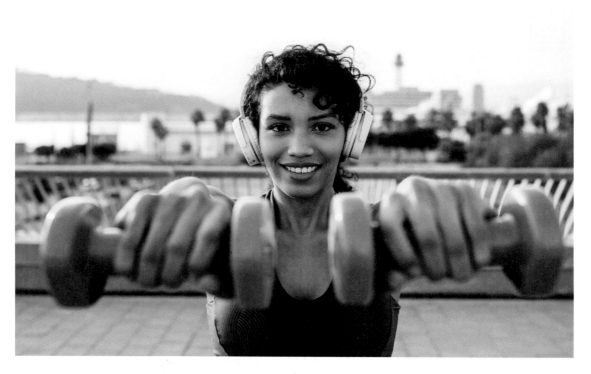

What to do after 28 days

Once you complete the four weeks of workouts, give yourself a big congratulations! Sticking to the plan for 28 days is something worth celebrating. Chances are you'll be feeling stronger, leaner, and more energized, so take some time to appreciate the progress you've made.

You'll also have laid a solid foundation for maintaining your healthy habits. To keep seeing results from resistance training, you'll need to make changes to the frequency, intensity, time, or types of exercises. Frequent changes will keep your body challenged, so it keeps getting stronger.

If you completed Program 1, you can up the ante by moving on to Program 2. (If any of the moves are still too difficult, substitute a move from the same day of Program 1.)

If you completed Program 2, try an amplified version of Program 1 by doubling the repetitions and circuit times. Do 4 sets of 16 in week 1, 8:00 circuits in week 2, 30:00 EMOMs in week 3, and 40:00 AMRAPs in week 4.

If you're ready to strike out on your own, continue to prioritize the Fab 4 and keep up a similar schedule with your weekly fitness plan. Alternate three days of resistance training and three days of cardiovascular training, and take one day of rest each week.

Remember, you have the knowledge it takes to sustain a Lift Light, Get Lean lifestyle. So continue your journey, and use the lessons you learn along the way to inspire others to improve their own health and wellness. Be the bridge.

CARDIOVASCULAR ENDURANCE WORKOUTS

Here are the options for aerobic exercise on Tuesdays, Thursdays, and Saturdays. Unlike the resistance exercises, which are assigned to specific days, you can choose which workout you do for each aerobic day. Remember to do the warmup on page 30 before each of these workouts.

Cardiovascular Endurance

Select **one** of these options on **Tuesdays, Thursdays, & Saturdays.**

RUCKING: Put your dumbbells in a backpack. Stand tall and walk/hike for 45 to 60 minutes.

THE BB INCLINE WALKING WORKOUT: Raise the grade (incline) by 1.0 on the treadmill every 3 minutes while walking at a challenging pace, then gradually reduce the incline. Walk for a total of 55 minutes.

2:1 POWER WALKING WORKOUT: Power walk (3.5 to 4.2 mph) for 2 minutes. Comfortably walk and hydrate for 1 minute. Repeat for a total of 10.

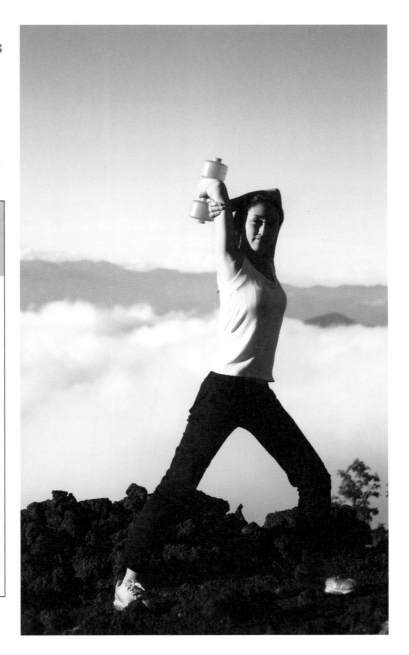

Exercise Library: Cardiovascular Endurance Workouts

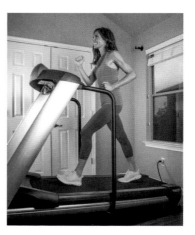

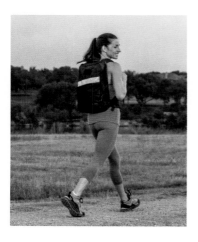

RUCKING

Rucking is the tried-and-true military practice of marching outdoors with a rucksack, or heavy-duty backpack, on your back. It's a low-impact aerobic exercise that utilizes added weights, so it boosts your cardiovascular fitness while toning your muscles, including your legs, glutes, back, and core. It also encourages you to stand taller and straighter as the straps of the sack pull your shoulders back. Who knew you could reap so many benefits just by slipping on a backpack and taking a walk?

You don't need to buy an official rucksack in order to ruck. A sturdy generic backpack that can hold your dumbbells or even a bag of rice will get the job done. (But if you prefer to use a true rucksack, American-made GORUCK rucksacks with ruck plates are the crème de la crème for durability and comfort.)

You can wear regular walking, running, or cross-training sneakers if you're rucking on pavement or grass. But it's a good idea to wear hiking boots if you'll be rucking on loose rocks. They've got better grip, so they'll reduce your risk for slipping and falling. And they'll be more comfortable for your feet and legs. Always bring more water than you think you'll need too, especially if it's hot out. Rucking can work up a sweat!

Here's the workout:

1. Put the filled rucksack/ backpack on your back. Find a hilly trail.

2. Walk at a challenging but comfortable pace for 45 to 60 minutes.

"THE BB" INCLINE WALKING WORKOUT

Yes, treadmill rhymes with dreadmill. But there's nothing to dread and much to gain from this low-impact incline walking workout for people of all fitness levels.

It's designed to challenge the heart, lungs, glutes, and legs. (As for the name, I've used it to train so many clients that many of them started calling it "The BB" after my initials!)

The BB starts off at a relatively low intensity and gets more challenging as the workout progresses. For that reason, I recommend starting just a wee bit below your usual brisk walking pace (for most people, between 3.5 and 4.2 mph) and decreasing your speed by 0.5 mph when you reach the 11% incline.

Be sure to wear supportive walking or running shoes for this workout. Walk with your foot strikes facing forward, not outward, and track your knees in the same direction as your toes. I like to pump my arms by my sides, but if you start to feel unsteady, grab the guardrails to regain your balance.

Here's the workout:

1. Spend three minutes at every whole-number gradient, 1 to 15. Because the difficulty of the hill becomes too much to bear at the starting cadence when you get to the 11% incline, you'll decrease the speed by 0.5 mph at that time.
2. After completing three minutes at 15% gradient, reduce the incline by 2% every minute.*

You can follow the chart to the right for a minute-by-minute breakdown.

*If you're new to exercise, only climb to 10% incline, then begin decreasing by 2% every minute thereafter. You may also need to reduce the speed recommendations by 0.5 mph.

*If you have a very strong aerobic base, consider increasing the speed by 0.5 mph (3.9 mph for 0 to 10% grade, 3.4% for 11 to 15% grade).

ELAPSED TIME (MIN.)	INCLINE %	PACE (MPH)
0	0%	3.4
3	1%	3.4
6	2%	3.4
9	3%	3.4
12	4%	3.4
15	5%	3.4
18	6%	3.4
21	7%	3.4
24	8%	3.4
27	9%	3.4
30	10%	3.4
33	11%	2.9
36	12%	2.9
39	13%	2.9
42	14%	2.9
45	15%	2.9
48	13%	2.9
49	11%	2.9
50	9%	3.4
51	7%	3.4
52	5%	3.4
53	3%	3.4
54	1%	3.4
55	0%	3.4

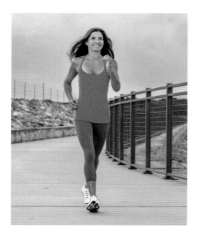

2:1 POWER WALKING WORKOUT

This is a high/low interval workout with a two-to-one ratio of hard work to recovery. During the high intervals, you'll walk at the fastest pace you can without transitioning to a jog. For most people, that's somewhere between 3.5 and 4.2 mph. (Avoid accelerating to a jog to keep this workout low-impact.) Follow the high interval with a leisurely walk, and repeat.

Wear supportive walking, running, or cross-training sneakers for this workout. Keep a water bottle with you and sip during your recovery periods.

Here's the workout:

1. **2:00** walk briskly at 3.5 to 4.2 miles per hour (or as fast as you can)
2. **1:00** walk slowly and prioritize recovery
3. Repeat for 10 rounds, for a total of 30 minutes

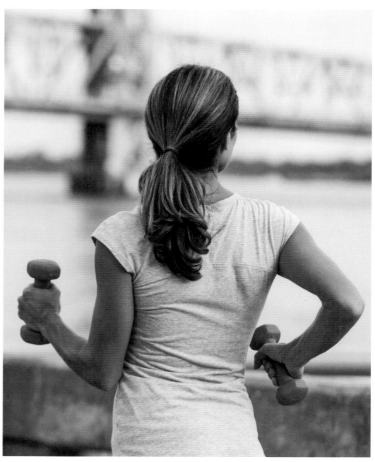

What you'll need

One set of light dumbbells is a must for this program. That said, having some other equipment on hand may make your workouts more comfortable and give you some extra versatility.

For Light Lifting

NEEDS

- One set of light hex-shaped dumbbells (see Pick the Right Weight on page 49). The hex shape is necessary to provide a stable base for moves like traveling bear planks, alternating renegade rows, bird dogs, plank to half pigeons, and hip bridge to crab rotations, which require holding weights while in a plank or crab position. If you don't have dumbbells, you can use your own body weight for those moves and then grab a sand- or pebbled-filled water bottle (water is too light) for everything else.

NICE-TO-HAVES

- Cross-training sneakers.
- Additional set of lighter dumbbells (3 to 5 pounds) for full body + core days.
- Yoga mat or padded rug, if you're following Program 2.
- Large water jug.
- Full-size towel and hand towel for wiping away sweat.
- Form-fitting clothes made of wicking fabric. (Baggy clothes can get in the way, especially in some of the swing moves.)

For Cardiovascular Endurance

NEEDS

- A backpack for carrying light dumbbells or a bag of rice, if you're doing the Rucking Workout.
- Walking or running sneakers.
- A treadmill, if you're performing the BB Incline Walking Workout (if you don't have a treadmill, you can select a different cardio workout).

NICE-TO-HAVES

- Hiking boots, if you're trekking on loose rocks or uneven terrain in the Rucking Workout.
- Sunscreen, if you're exercising outdoors.
- A tactical backpack or rucksack, if you're performing the Rucking Workout. These types of backpacks are more comfortable on your back, hips, chest, and shoulders for rucking.

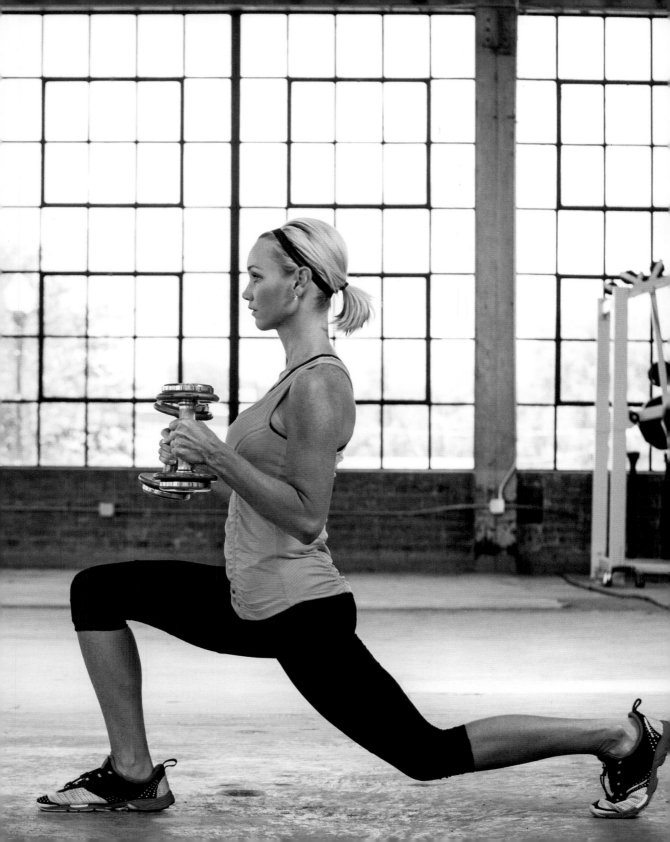

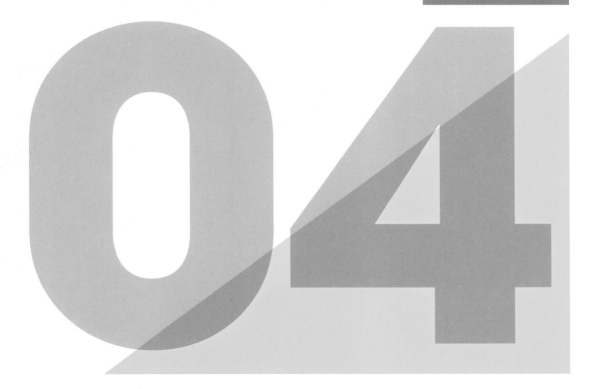

WEEKLY WORKOUTS

Now that you know how the plan works and have chosen which of the two programs you want to follow, spend some time getting to know the exercises you'll be performing. Here you'll find photos and step-by-step instructions for each exercise, plus modifications for some of the more challenging moves.

PROGRAM 1

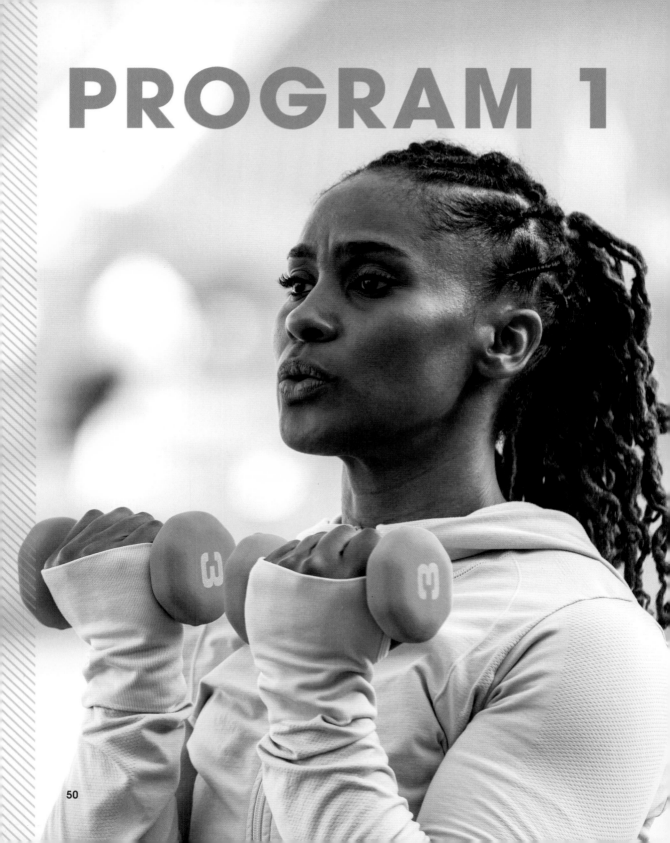

Habit Tracker

Recording your progress is a great way to stay motivated on the plan and see just how far you've come. Use this daily tracker to document your journey by putting a checkmark in the boxes for each day you complete the habit listed.

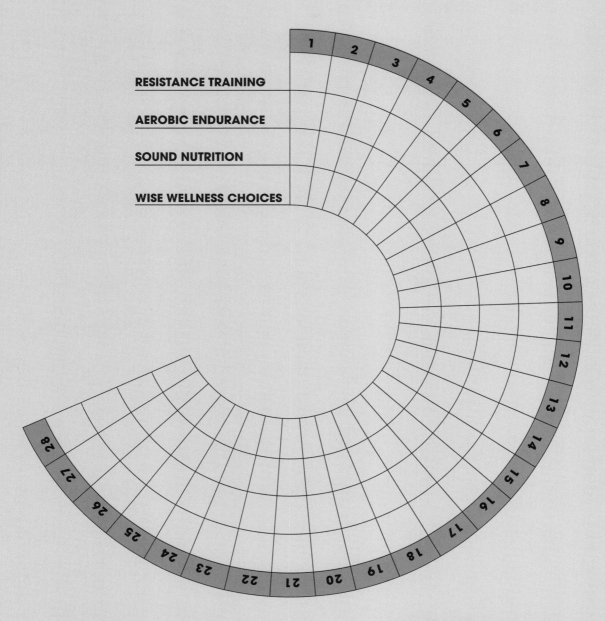

RESISTANCE TRAINING

AEROBIC ENDURANCE

SOUND NUTRITION

WISE WELLNESS CHOICES

Week 1 At-A-Glance

This week do 16 reps of each exercise for 2 sets.

	WORKOUT
MONDAY	Lower-Body Moves (p. 53)
TUESDAY	Cardio
WEDNESDAY	Upper-Body Moves (p. 54)
THURSDAY	Cardio
FRIDAY	Full-Body and Core (p. 55)
SATURDAY	Cardio
SUNDAY	Rest

Tip of the Week

DOCUMENT YOUR HARD WORK. One of the best ways to establish new habits is writing down what you accomplish. So we've provided space for you to record the amount of weight you used for your workout, notes on how the session felt, and your wellness and nutrition wins. We've also included a 28-day habit tracker for each program (pages 51 and 87), so you can check off your daily Fab 4 achievements. Because is there anything as instantly rewarding as checking off your to-do's? Research backs us up: Gallup's CliftonStrengths assessment shows that people who rank high as "Achievers" thrive by starting each day with a checklist. Follow the plan to a tee, and your habit tracker will have three check marks Monday through Saturday (nutrition, wellness, and resistance training or aerobic endurance), and two on Sunday, your rest day (nutrition and wellness).

LOWER-BODY MOVES

	EXERCISE	WORK	SETS	WEIGHT	NOTES
	Front Two-Handed Swings (p. 68)	16 Reps	2		
	Forward Lunges (p. 69)	16 Reps	2		
	Curtsy Lunges (p. 70)	16 Reps	2		
	Lateral Lunges (p. 71)	16 Reps	2		
	Back Lunges (p. 72)	16 Reps	2		
	Sumo Squats (p. 73)	16 Reps	2		

UPPER-BODY MOVES

	EXERCISE	WORK	SETS	WEIGHT	NOTES
	High Pulls (p. 74)	**16 Reps**	**2**		
	Pec Deck to Overhead Presses (p. 75)	**16 Reps**	**2**		
	Reverse Flys (p. 76)	**16 Reps**	**2**		
	Alternating MAC Raises (p. 77)	**16 Reps**	**2**		
	Supinated Rows (a.k.a., Biceps Rows) (p. 78)	**16 Reps**	**2**		
	Triceps Kickbacks (p. 79)	**16 Reps**	**2**		

FULL BODY AND CORE

	EXERCISE	WORK	SETS	WEIGHT	NOTES
	Squat to Presses (p. 80)	16 Reps	2		
	Right Leg Lunge Back to Biceps Curls (p. 81)	16 Reps	2		
	Left Leg Lunge Back to Overhead Triceps Extensions (p.82)	16 Reps	2		
	Dead Lift to Scaptions (p. 83)	16 Reps	2		
	Sumo Squat to Upright Rows (p. 84)	16 Reps	2		
	Hip Abduction to Lateral Shoulder Raises (p.85)	16 Reps	2		

Week 2 At-A-Glance

This week do 40 seconds of each exercise for 2 sets. If needed, rest between sets and resume when you feel recovered.

	WORKOUT
MONDAY	**Lower-Body Moves (p. 57)**
TUESDAY	**Cardio**
WEDNESDAY	**Upper-Body Moves (p. 58)**
THURSDAY	**Cardio**
FRIDAY	**Full-Body and Core (p. 59)**
SATURDAY	**Cardio**
SUNDAY	**Rest**

Tip of the Week

EXECUTE THE PERFECT SWING. When done right, swings can be incredibly effective. However, they can be tricky to nail as they're a little bit of an optical illusion—they can look similar to the front shoulder raises you might've done a hundred times before. But the physics involved with a swing are different from the controlled effort of a front shoulder raise. This is more like tetherball, where the ball swings on a rope that hangs from a pole. The force driving the ball (the dumbbell) out is the push that sends it swinging, not the rope (your arms). Likewise, with swings, the shoulders are not lifting the weight. Your strong hip thrust is the force, or push, that drives the weight out. That hip thrust is powered by the posterior chain (glutes, hamstrings, and back). Focus on keeping your back flat and hinging your hips back, then squeezing your glutes and tightening your abs at the top to stop the motion when your shoulders are over your hips and you're standing perfectly erect.

LOWER-BODY MOVES

	EXERCISE	WORK	SETS	WEIGHT	NOTES
	Front Two-Handed Swings (p. 68)	40 sec.	2		
	Forward Lunges (p. 69)	40 sec.	2		
	Curtsy Lunges (p. 70)	40 sec.	2		
	Lateral Lunges (p. 71)	40 sec.	2		
	Back Lunges (p. 72)	40 sec.	2		
	Sumo Squats (p. 73)	40 sec.	2		

UPPER-BODY MOVES

	EXERCISE	WORK	SETS	WEIGHT	NOTES
	High Pulls (p. 74)	40 sec.	2		
	Pec Deck to Overhead Presses (p. 75)	40 sec.	2		
	Reverse Flys (p. 76)	40 sec.	2		
	Alternating MAC Raises (p. 77)	40 sec.	2		
	Supinated Rows (a.k.a., Biceps Rows) (p. 78)	40 sec.	2		
	Triceps Kickbacks (p. 79)	40 sec.	2		

FULL BODY AND CORE

	EXERCISE	WORK	SETS	WEIGHT	NOTES
	Squat to Presses (p. 80)	40 sec.	2		
	Right Leg Lunge Back to Biceps Curls (p. 81)	40 sec.	2		
	Left Leg Lunge Back to Overhead Triceps Extensions (p. 82)	40 sec.	2		
	Dead Lift to Scaptions (p. 83)	40 sec.	2		
	Sumo Squat to Upright Rows (p. 84)	40 sec.	2		
	Hip Abduction to Lateral Shoulder Raises (p. 85)	40 sec.	2		

Week 3 At-A-Glance

This week you'll do the moves EMOM-style (every minute on the minute). Begin each exercise at the start of a minute. Perform 2 reps, then use the remaining time in the minute as your rest. Repeat for a total of 15 minutes.

	WORKOUT
MONDAY	**Lower-Body Moves (p. 61)**
TUESDAY	Cardio
WEDNESDAY	**Upper-Body Moves (p. 62)**
THURSDAY	Cardio
FRIDAY	**Full-Body and Core (p. 63)**
SATURDAY	Cardio
SUNDAY	Rest

Tip of the Week

BOOST WILLPOWER BY REMEMBERING YOUR "WHY." Maybe you started this program chock-full of willpower. How's that going for you? Willpower is like the determination a child has at the start of a fun run—she shoots out of the gate like it's an Olympic track race. But after an initial sprint, she's toast. The three-week mark in this program is like the end of that sprint. Life is long. To help clients understand what sets temporary change apart from life-long habits, I like to use the Stages of Change model, developed by psychotherapists James Prochaska and Carlo Di Clemente. The model identifies a sequence of five stages—precontemplation, contemplation, preparation, action, and maintenance—that people move through as they adopt a new habit. Buying this book means you've leapfrogged right into the action stage—but if you feel an ebb in motivation, back up and remember those prior stages. Take a moment to journal about why you purchased the book and to note your goals. That can serve as a reminder as you continue to build your workout and nutrition habits, then maintain them.

LOWER-BODY MOVES

	EXERCISE	WORK	SETS	WEIGHT	NOTES
	Front Two-Handed Swings (p. 68)	2 Reps	15 min. EMOM		
	Forward Lunges (p. 69)	2 Reps	15 min. EMOM		
	Curtsy Lunges (p. 70)	2 Reps	15 min. EMOM		
	Lateral Lunges (p. 71)	2 Reps	15 min. EMOM		
	Back Lunges (p. 72)	2 Reps	15 min. EMOM		
	Sumo Squats (p. 73)	2 Reps	15 min. EMOM		

UPPER-BODY MOVES

	EXERCISE	WORK	SETS	WEIGHT	NOTES
	High Pulls (p. 74)	2 Reps	15 min. EMOM		
	Pec Deck to Overhead Presses (p. 75)	2 Reps	15 min. EMOM		
	Reverse Flys (p. 76)	2 Reps	15 min. EMOM		
	Alternating MAC Raises (p. 77)	2 Reps	15 min. EMOM		
	Supinated Rows (a.k.a., Biceps Rows) (p. 78)	2 Reps	15 min. EMOM		
	Triceps Kickbacks (p. 79)	2 Reps	15 min. EMOM		

FULL BODY AND CORE

	EXERCISE	WORK	SETS	WEIGHT	NOTES
	Squat to Presses (p. 80)	2 Reps	15 min. EMOM		
	Right Leg Lunge Back to Biceps Curls (p. 81)	2 Reps	15 min. EMOM		
	Left Leg Lunge Back to Overhead Triceps Extensions (p. 82)	2 Reps	15 min. EMOM		
	Dead Lift to Scaptions (p. 83)	2 Reps	15 min. EMOM		
	Sumo Squat to Upright Rows (p. 84)	2 Reps	15 min. EMOM		
	Hip Abduction to Lateral Shoulder Raises (p. 85)	2 Reps	15 min. EMOM		

Week 4 At-A-Glance

This week you'll do the moves AMRAP-style (as many rounds as possible). Do 4 reps of each exercise with 10 seconds of rest after completing all moves. Repeat for as many rounds as possible in 20 minutes.

	WORKOUT
MONDAY	Lower-Body Moves (p. 65)
TUESDAY	Cardio
WEDNESDAY	Upper-Body Moves (p. 66)
THURSDAY	Cardio
FRIDAY	Full-Body and Core (p. 67)
SATURDAY	Cardio
SUNDAY	Rest

Tip of the Week

TRY SOME NEW FIBER-FILLED FOODS. By this point, you may be looking to shake up what's on your plate, but don't forget about fiber. High-fiber foods lower blood sugar. Furthermore, such foods trigger weight loss while keeping you feeling full. Listen to how well it worked for one test panel participant, Kelly. "I did the high-protein/low-carb ritual for years, and my weight would be a roller coaster. I was tired and always in a mental fog. This high-fiber approach is giving my body the right nutrients, I'm losing weight, and I'm actually feeling healthy again." Here are some delicious ways to boost your fiber from whole foods: ¼ cup dry steel-cut oats, cooked, with one chopped apple for breakfast (10 g of fiber—this option doubles the fiber you'd get from just a bowl of rolled oats!); a hearty bowl of lentil soup for lunch (12 g of fiber in 1 cup); a cup of steamed broccoli and a cup of Brussels sprouts with your dinner (8 g of fiber, collectively); and a cup of rasp-berries for dessert (8 g of fiber).

LOWER-BODY MOVES

	EXERCISE	WORK	SETS	WEIGHT	NOTES
	Front Two-Handed Swings (p. 68)	4 Reps	20 min. AMRAP		
	Forward Lunges (p. 69)	4 Reps	20 min. AMRAP		
	Curtsy Lunges (p. 70)	4 Reps	20 min. AMRAP		
	Lateral Lunges (p. 71)	4 Reps	20 min. AMRAP		
	Back Lunges (p. 72)	4 Reps	20 min. AMRAP		
	Sumo Squats (p. 73)	4 Reps	20 min. AMRAP		

UPPER-BODY MOVES

	EXERCISE	WORK	SETS	WEIGHT	NOTES
	High Pulls (p. 74)	4 Reps	20 min. AMRAP		
	Pec Deck to Overhead Presses (p. 75)	4 Reps	20 min. AMRAP		
	Reverse Flys (p. 76)	4 Reps	20 min. AMRAP		
	Alternating MAC Raises (p. 77)	4 Reps	20 min. AMRAP		
	Supinated Rows (a.k.a., Biceps Rows) (p. 78)	4 Reps	20 min. AMRAP		
	Triceps Kickbacks (p. 79)	4 Reps	20 min. AMRAP		

FULL BODY AND CORE

	EXERCISE	WORK	SETS	WEIGHT	NOTES
	Squat to Presses (p. 80)	4 Reps	20 min. AMRAP		
	Right Leg Lunge Back to Biceps Curls (p. 81)	4 Reps	20 min. AMRAP		
	Left Leg Lunge Back to Overhead Triceps Extensions (p.82)	4 Reps	20 min. AMRAP		
	Dead Lift to Scaptions (p. 83)	4 Reps	20 min. AMRAP		
	Sumo Squat to Upright Rows (p. 84)	4 Reps	20 min. AMRAP		
	Hip Abduction to Lateral Shoulder Raises (p.85)	4 Reps	20 min. AMRAP		

LOWER-BODY MOVES

FRONT TWO-HANDED SWINGS

WHAT IT WORKS

Glutes, hamstrings, lower back, heart, and lungs

HOW TO DO IT

SETUP Hold a dumbbell in each hand at your thighs. Stand erect with shoulders over hips and legs slightly wider than hip-width apart, toes facing forward.

STEP 1 Hinge at your hips, driving the dumbbells between your legs up to the tops of your inner thighs.

STEP 2 Powerfully push your hips forward, propelling the weights forward to shoulder height. Allow gravity to take charge and arc the weights back to the starting position. That's 1 rep.

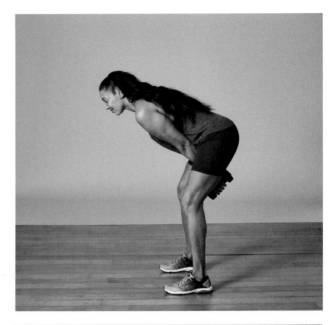

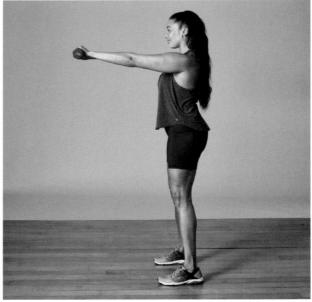

FORWARD LUNGES

WHAT IT WORKS

Quadriceps and glutes

HOW TO DO IT

SETUP Stand erect and hold a dumbbell in each hand.

STEP 1 Lunge forward with one foot.

STEP 2 Push off on your front foot to return to the starting position. Repeat on the opposite leg. That's 1 rep.

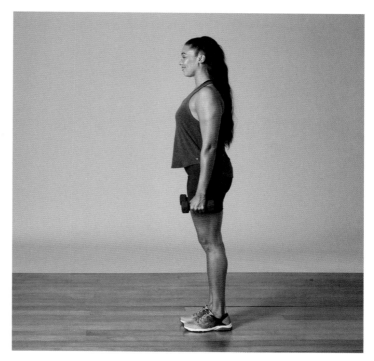

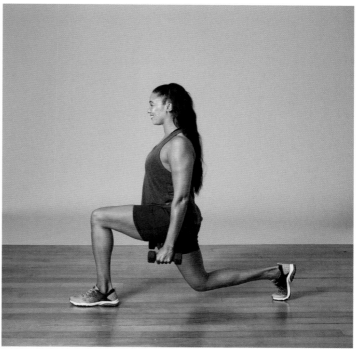

CURTSY LUNGES

WHAT IT WORKS

Sides of the glutes and
quadriceps

HOW TO DO IT

SETUP Stand erect with your
feet hip-width apart and arms by
your sides, holding a dumbbell
in each hand.

STEP 1 Stay planted on one foot.
Extend your other foot behind
you, putting it on the floor in
line with the outside of your front
foot, as if you were beginning
a curtsy. Bend your knees and
lower your back shin so it
hovers right above the floor. Hold
momentarily.

STEP 2 Push off your back leg
to return to the starting position.
Repeat on the opposite leg.
That's 1 rep.

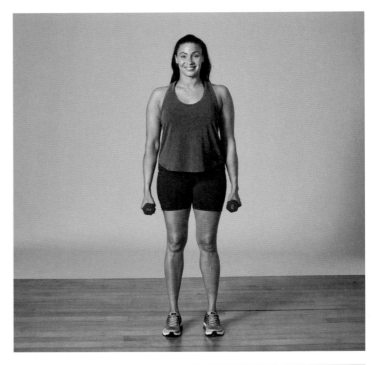

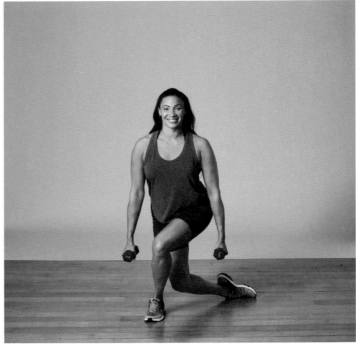

LATERAL LUNGES

WHAT IT WORKS

Sides of the glutes and outer thighs

HOW TO DO IT

SETUP Stand with your feet hip-width apart and arms by your sides, holding a dumbbell in each hand.

STEP 1 Step to the side with one leg. Shift your hips out and back, bending the working leg. Lower the dumbbells toward your foot. Keep your chest open, facing forward.

STEP 2 Push off with the foot of the bent leg to propel yourself back to the starting position. Repeat on the opposite side. That's 1 rep.

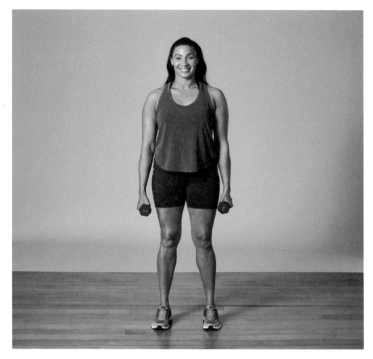

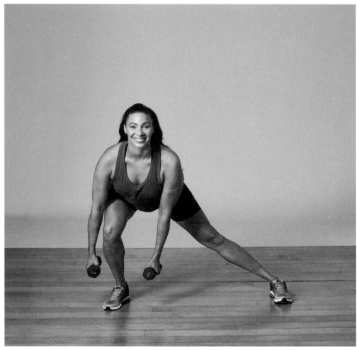

BACK LUNGES

WHAT IT WORKS

Quadriceps and glutes

HOW TO DO IT

SETUP Stand tall with your feet hip-width apart and arms by your sides, holding a dumbbell in each hand.

STEP 1 Step one foot back into a lunge.

STEP 2 Push off on your back foot to return to standing. Repeat on the opposite leg. That's 1 rep.

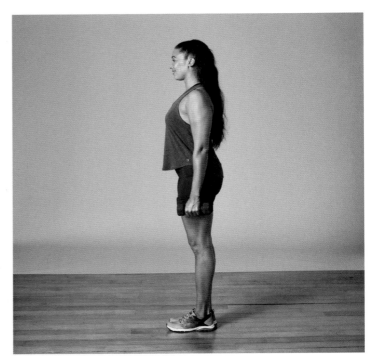

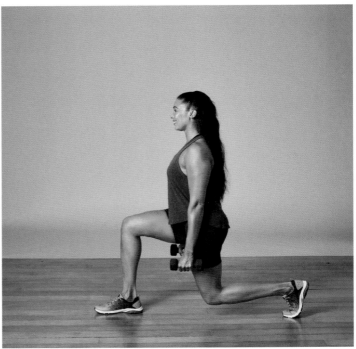

SUMO SQUATS

WHAT IT WORKS

Glutes, quadriceps, and inner thighs

HOW TO DO IT

SETUP Stand erect with your feet wider than hip-width apart and toes pointing out to the sides. Hold a dumbbell in each hand, arms dangling in front of your body.

STEP 1 Keeping your chest lifted, bend your knees to sink into a squat. Drop as low as you can, optimally until your thighs are parallel to the floor. Hold momentarily.

STEP 2 Driving from your heels, return to the starting position, squeezing your inner thighs and tightening your tush. That's 1 rep.

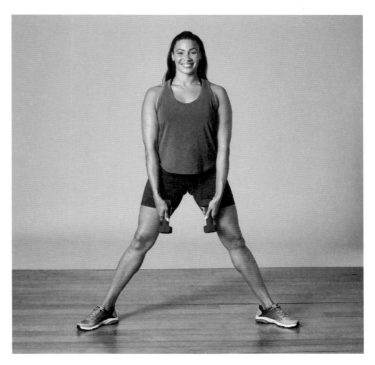

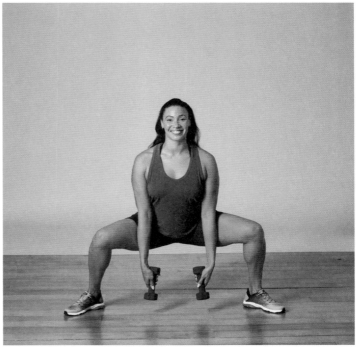

UPPER-BODY MOVES

HIGH PULLS

WHAT IT WORKS

Glutes, hamstrings, lower back, upper back, backs of the shoulders, and posture

HOW TO DO IT

SETUP Hold a dumbbell in each hand. Stand erect with your shoulders over your hips and legs slightly wider than hip-width apart, toes facing forward.

STEP 1 Hinge at your hips, driving the dumbbells between your legs up to the tops of your inner thighs.

STEP 2 Powerfully push your hips forward, propelling the weights forward, then engage your upper-body strength to pull the weights in toward your shoulders with elbows out. Punch your arms out and drop the weights in an arc to return to starting position. That's 1 rep.

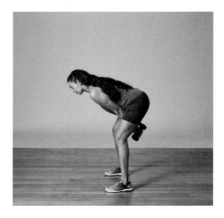

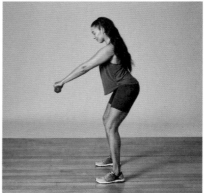

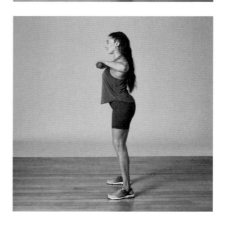

PEC DECK TO OVERHEAD PRESSES

WHAT IT WORKS

Chest and shoulders

HOW TO DO IT

SETUP Stand erect with your shoulders over your hips and your legs slightly more than hip-width apart, toes facing forward. Hold a dumbbell in each hand with arms bent to 90 degrees, elbows at shoulder height.

STEP 1 Draw your elbows together to bring your forearms together in front of your face. Hold momentarily, then return to starting position.

STEP 2 Maintaining good posture, press your arms overhead so your wrists, elbows, and shoulders are aligned. Hold momentarily, then return to starting position. That's 1 rep.

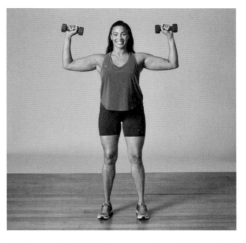

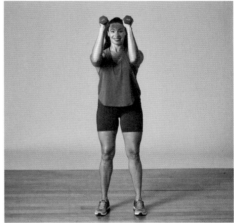

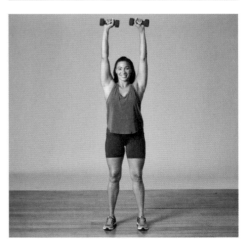

REVERSE FLYS

WHAT IT WORKS

Backs of the shoulders
and upper back

HOW TO DO IT

SETUP Hold a dumbbell in each
hand. Engage your core and tip
forward at your hips, maintaining
a flat back. Dangle your arms
below your chest.

STEP 1 Raise your knuckles
toward the ceiling with elbows
barely bent. Hold momentarily.

STEP 2 Slowly lower your arms
to touch the dumbbells in front of
your chest. That's 1 rep.

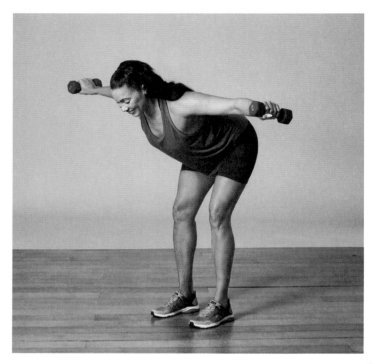

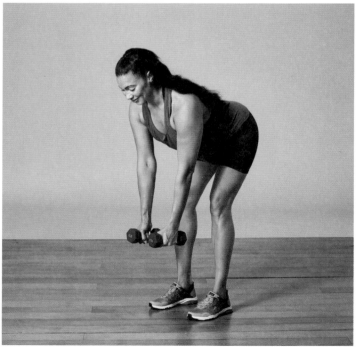

ALTERNATING MAC RAISES

WHAT IT WORKS

Fronts and sides of the shoulders

HOW TO DO IT

SETUP Stand erect with shoulders over hips and legs slightly more than hip-width apart, toes facing forward. Hold a dumbbell in each hand in front of your thighs.

STEP 1 Extend one arm straight in front of you. Bend the other elbow to 90 degrees as you lift the weight. Hold momentarily, then return to starting position.

STEP 2 Repeat on the opposite side. That's 1 rep.

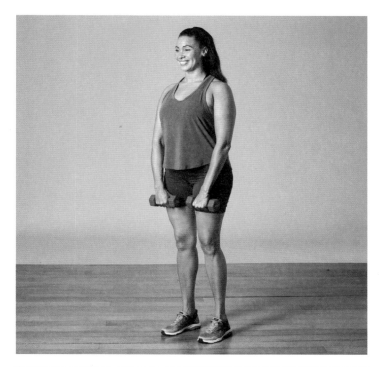

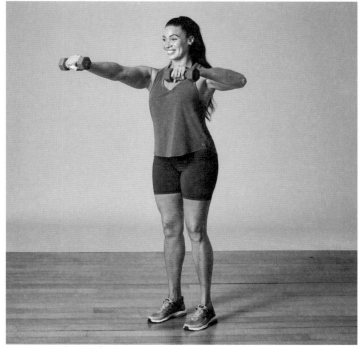

SUPINATED ROWS (A.K.A., BICEPS ROWS)

WHAT IT WORKS

Back and biceps

HOW TO DO IT

SETUP With a dumbbell in each hand, stand with your legs slightly wider than hip-width apart, knees slightly bent. Engage your core to maintain a flat back as you tip forward at your hips to bring your back parallel to the floor (like the top of a table). Let your arms hang in front of you, and turn your arms so your palms face forward.

STEP 1 Pull your elbows up, straight past your ribcage, drawing the dumbbells to touch your abdomen. Hold momentarily. Be sure to keep your palms facing forward the entire time to keep the biceps muscles as engaged as possible.

STEP 2 Slowly return the weights to starting position. That's 1 rep.

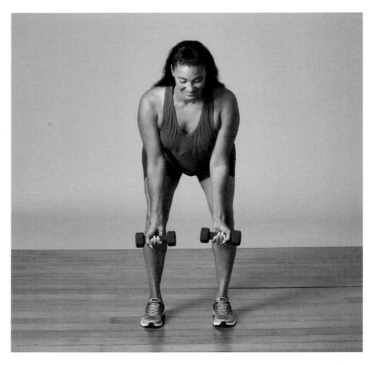

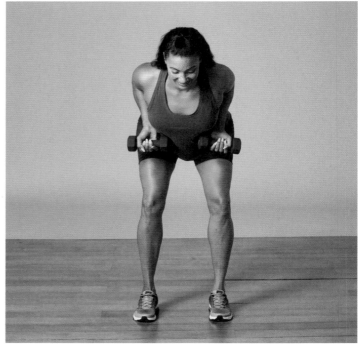

TRICEPS KICKBACKS

WHAT IT WORKS

Triceps

HOW TO DO IT

SETUP Hold a dumbbell in each hand. Engage your core and hinge forward at your hips, maintaining a flat back. Pull your elbows into your low ribs and hold them steady there.

STEP 1 Extend your elbows and reach the dumbbells straight behind your hips. Hold momentarily.

STEP 2 Bend your elbows and bring the dumbbells back in, keeping them in line with your shoulders. That's 1 rep.

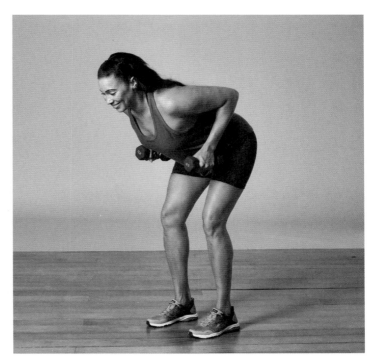

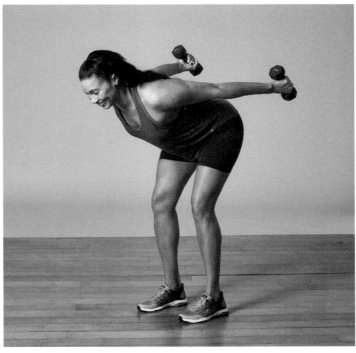

FULL BODY AND CORE

SQUAT TO PRESSES

WHAT IT WORKS

Quadriceps, glutes, core, and shoulders

HOW TO DO IT

SETUP Stand with your shoulders over your hips and your legs slightly more than hip-width apart, toes facing forward. Rack your dumbbells so that they are level with your collarbones.

STEP 1 Keeping your chest lifted and spine tall, bend your knees and sink your hips into a squat, tracking your knees in the same direction as your toes. Drop as low as you can, optimally deeper than 90 degrees. Hold momentarily.

STEP 2 Squeeze your glutes and rise to starting position.

STEP 3 Keeping your legs and core motionless, raise the dumbbells overhead so your wrists are straight over your shoulders.

STEP 4 Return to starting position with dumbbells racked at your collarbones. That's 1 rep.

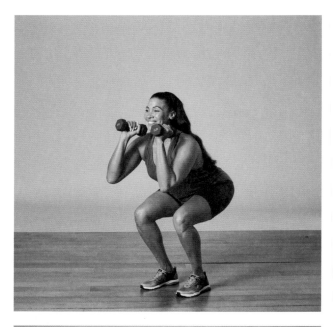

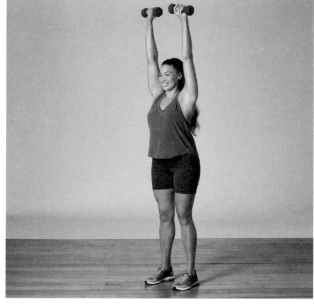

RIGHT LEG LUNGE BACK TO BICEPS CURLS

WHAT IT WORKS

Quadriceps, glutes, core, biceps, and balance

HOW TO DO IT

SETUP Hold a dumbbell in each hand, arms by your sides. Stand erect with your shoulders over your hips and your legs hip-width apart, toes facing forward.

STEP 1 Step your right foot back into a deep lunge.

STEP 2 Squeeze your glutes and return your back foot to the setup position, keeping the majority of your weight on the supporting leg to challenge your balance.

STEP 3 Bend your elbows and draw the dumbbells toward your shoulders in a biceps curl.

STEP 4 Extend your elbows to return to starting position. That's 1 rep.

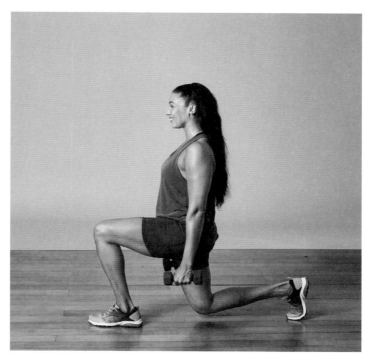

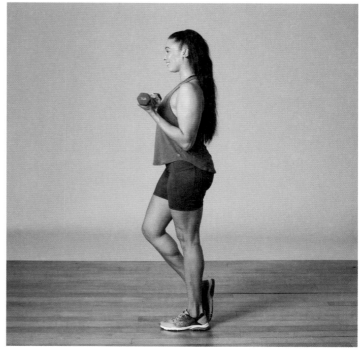

LEFT LEG LUNGE BACK TO OVERHEAD TRICEPS EXTENSIONS

WHAT IT WORKS

Quadriceps, glutes, core, shoulders, triceps, and balance

HOW TO DO IT

SETUP Hold a dumbbell in each hand, arms by your sides. Stand erect with your shoulders over your hips and your feet hip-width apart, toes facing forward.

STEP 1 Step your left foot back into a deep lunge.

STEP 2 Squeeze your glutes and return your back foot to the setup position, keeping the majority of your weight on the supporting leg to challenge your balance.

STEP 3 Raise your arms above your head so they're close to your ears. Bend your elbows and lower the dumbbells behind your head until they touch (or nearly touch) your shoulders. Keep your elbows pointing forward and not out to the sides.

STEP 4 Extend both elbows to return the dumbbells overhead, then lower them to the setup position. That's 1 rep.

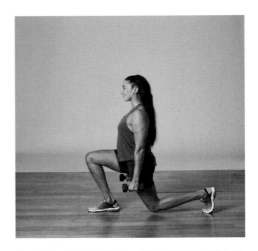

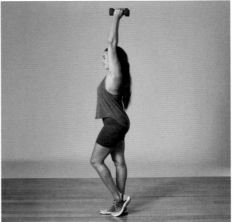

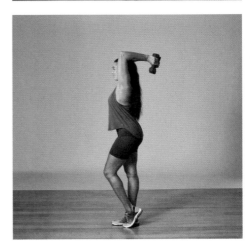

DEAD LIFT TO SCAPTIONS

WHAT IT WORKS

Hamstrings, lower back, glutes, core, upper back, and backs of the shoulders

HOW TO DO IT

SETUP Hold a dumbbell in each hand, arms dangling in front of your body. Stand erect with your shoulders over your hips and your feet hip-width apart, toes facing forward.

STEP 1 Hinge at your hips and glide the dumbbells down the fronts of your thighs. Maintain just a tiny bend in your knees. Keep your back flat.

STEP 2 Squeeze your glutes, push through both feet, and rise up to starting position.

STEP 3 Without bending your arms, lift them up to form a "V" while squeezing your upper back muscles in together tightly. Hold momentarily.

STEP 4 Release the contraction in your upper back and return your arms to starting position. That's 1 rep.

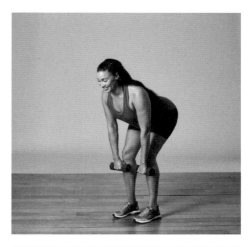

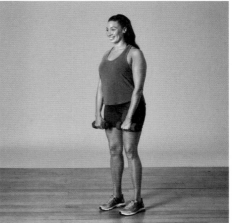

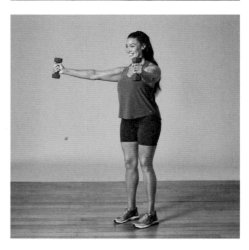

SUMO SQUAT TO UPRIGHT ROWS

WHAT IT WORKS

Quadriceps, glutes, inner thighs, core,
and shoulders

HOW TO DO IT

SETUP Stand erect with your feet more than
hip-width apart and toes pointing out to the sides.
Hold a dumbbell in each hand, arms dangling
in front of your body.

STEP 1 Keeping your chest lifted, bend your knees
and sink into a squat. Drop as low as you can,
optimally until your thighs are parallel to the floor.
Hold momentarily.

STEP 2 Driving from your heels, return to the
starting position, squeezing your inner thighs and
tightening your tush.

STEP 3 Pull both dumbbells up your torso,
winging your elbows out to the sides. Finish
with your elbows slightly below shoulder
height with the dumbbells at your sternum.

STEP 4 Lower the dumbbells down your torso to
return to starting position. That's 1 rep.

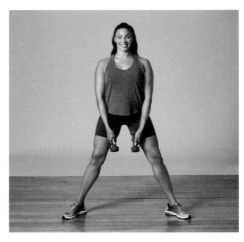
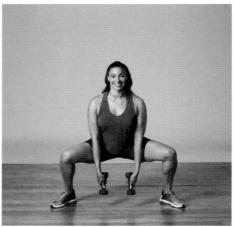
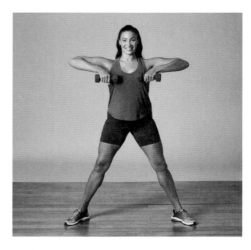

HIP ABDUCTION TO LATERAL SHOULDER RAISES

WHAT IT WORKS

Sides of the glutes, outer thighs, core, and sides of the shoulders

HOW TO DO IT

SETUP Hold a dumbbell in each hand, resting your hands and the weights on your outer thighs. Stand erect with your shoulders over your hips and your legs hip-width apart, toes facing forward.

STEP 1 Flex one foot and lift that leg out to the side, away from the midline of the body.

STEP 2 Return the leg to the setup position.

STEP 3 Keep your arms straight and lift the dumbbells up and away from your body until you make a "T" shape. Hold momentarily.

STEP 4 Slowly lower the dumbbells back to your outer thighs. That's 1 rep. Repeat on the opposite side.

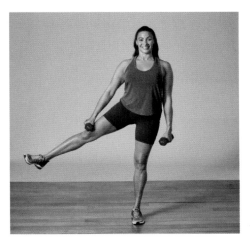

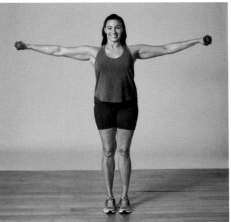

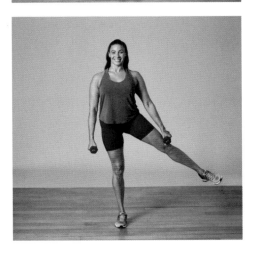

PROGRAM 2

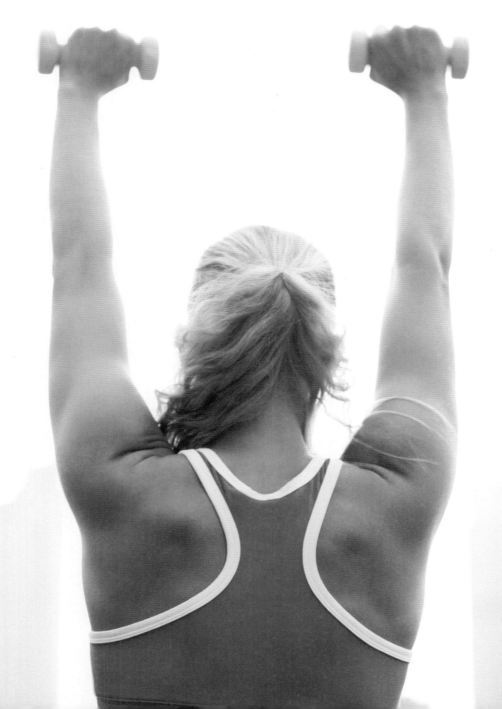

Habit Tracker

Recording your progress is a great way to stay motivated on the plan and see just how far you've come. Use this daily tracker to document your journey by putting a checkmark in the boxes for each day you complete the habit listed.

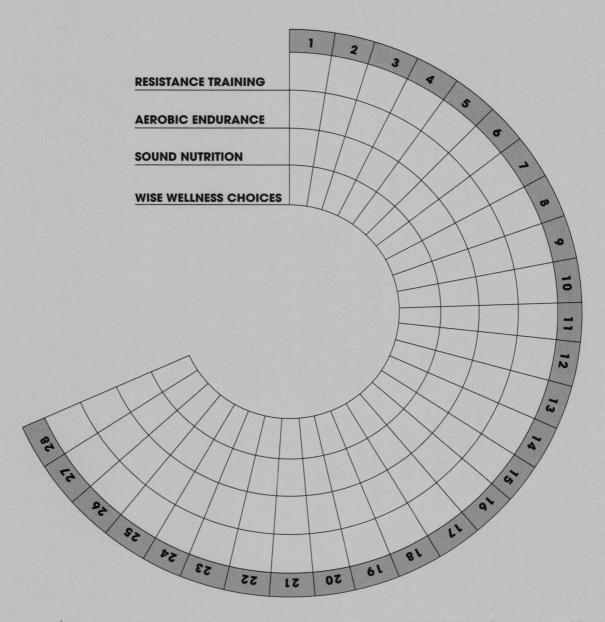

RESISTANCE TRAINING

AEROBIC ENDURANCE

SOUND NUTRITION

WISE WELLNESS CHOICES

Week 1 At-A-Glance

This week do 16 reps of each exercise for 2 sets.

	WORKOUT
MONDAY	**Lower-Body Moves (p. 89)**
TUESDAY	Cardio
WEDNESDAY	**Upper-Body Moves (p. 90)**
THURSDAY	Cardio
FRIDAY	**Full-Body and Core (p. 91)**
SATURDAY	Cardio
SUNDAY	Rest

Tip of the Week

MAKE MOBILITY A PRIORITY.
"Mobility" means the ability to move freely and easily. Although it isn't directly associated with weight loss, you can't tone what you can't train. You want a perky butt? You need to squat deep. And to squat deep, you need mobility. That's why I built mobility into your Friday workouts—it may catch you by surprise! All other workouts in this book are performed standing. But on Friday, you'll be on the floor, doing assorted prone (belly down) and supine (belly up) moves. You'll also do tons of mobility work, especially for the hips. Hip mobility is super important because when the glutes get tight, the hips get less mobile—and cause more pain. That's a real shame because the hips should be among the most mobile parts of your whole body (second only to shoulders)! Exercises in this workout, like plank to half pigeon and hip bridge to crab rotation, will help to improve the range of motion in your hips, unlock tight glutes, and improve core strength.

LOWER-BODY MOVES

	EXERCISE	WORK	SETS	WEIGHT	NOTES
	Alternating Swings (p. 104)	16 Reps	2		
	Right Lunge Back with Dumbbell Swing Backs (p. 105)	16 Reps	2		
	Right Skater to Balance Holds (p. 106)	16 Reps	2		
	Rainbow Lunges (p. 107)	16 Reps	2		
	Left Lunge Back with Dumbbell Swing Backs (p. 105)	16 Reps	2		
	Left Skater to Balance Holds (p. 106)	16 Reps	2		

UPPER-BODY MOVES

	EXERCISE	WORK	SETS	WEIGHT	NOTES
	American Swings (p. 104)	16 Reps	2		
	ISO Biceps Hold at 90 Degrees with Alternating Lunge Backs (p. 109)	16 Reps	2		
	Reciprocal Bent-Over Rows (a.k.a., Milk the Cow) (p. 110)	16 Reps	2		
	Overhead Triceps Extensions (p. 111)	16 Reps	2		
	Arnold Presses (p. 112)	16 Reps	2		
	90-Degree Lateral Raises (p. 113)	16 Reps	2		

FULL BODY AND CORE

	EXERCISE	WORK	SETS	WEIGHT	NOTES
	Traveling Bear Planks (p. 114)	16 Reps	2		
	Alternating Renegade Rows (p. 115)	16 Reps	2		
	Bird Dogs (p. 116)	16 Reps	2		
	Plank to Half Pigeons (Alternating) (p. 117)	16 Reps	2		
	Hip Bridge to Crab Rotations (p. 118)	16 Reps	2		
	Flutter Kicks with Arms over Shoulders (p. 119)	16 Reps	2		

Week 2 At-A-Glance

This week do 40 seconds of each exercise for 2 sets. If needed, rest between sets and resume when you feel recovered.

	WORKOUT
MONDAY	Lower-Body Moves (p. 93)
TUESDAY	Cardio
WEDNESDAY	Upper-Body Moves (p. 94)
THURSDAY	Cardio
FRIDAY	Full-Body and Core (p. 95)
SATURDAY	Cardio
SUNDAY	Rest

Tip of the Week

EMBRACE THAT OUT-OF-BREATH FEELING. If you find yourself panting your way through the Monday workout in Program 2, you're not the only one. Jen Upah, one of the women in our test panel, asked, "Should I be feeling so much cardio in this workout?" The answer is yes. Because you are performing agility exercises and moving in different directions with moves like Skater to Balance Holds and Rainbow Lunges, your heart rate will climb. You will improve your athleticism, balance, and mobility. This workout will also strengthen your glutes, quadriceps, adductors, and hamstrings. You'll be racking up muscular endurance gains. And it's not "either/or" here. You get both! This workout takes your body through sagittal, frontal, and transverse planes and adds drills that are sports-skills applicable. But don't get so gung ho into sports mode that you move too rapidly. As you go through these intermediate/advanced moves, keep in mind that execution with precision and full range of motion is the goal.

LOWER-BODY MOVES

	EXERCISE	WORK	SETS	WEIGHT	NOTES
	Alternating Swings (p. 104)	40 sec.	2		
	Right Lunge Back with Dumbbell Swing Backs (p. 105)	40 sec.	2		
	Right Skater to Balance Holds (p. 106)	40 sec.	2		
	Rainbow Lunges (p. 107)	40 sec.	2		
	Left Lunge Back with Dumbbell Swing Backs (p. 105)	40 sec.	2		
	Left Skater to Balance Holds (p. 106)	40 sec.	2		

UPPER-BODY MOVES

	EXERCISE	WORK	SETS	WEIGHT	NOTES
	American Swings (p. 104)	**40 sec.**	**2**		
	ISO Biceps Hold at 90 Degrees with Alternating Lunge Backs (p. 109)	**40 sec.**	**2**		
	Reciprocal Bent-Over Rows (a.k.a., Milk the Cow) (p. 110)	**40 sec.**	**2**		
	Overhead Triceps Extensions (p. 111)	**40 sec.**	**2**		
	Arnold Presses (p. 112)	**40 sec.**	**2**		
	90-Degree Lateral Raises (p. 113)	**40 sec.**	**2**		

FULL BODY AND CORE

	EXERCISE	WORK	SETS	WEIGHT	NOTES
	Traveling Bear Planks (p. 114)	40 sec.	2		
	Alternating Renegade Rows (p. 115)	40 sec.	2		
	Bird Dogs (p. 116)	40 sec.	2		
	Plank to Half Pigeons (Alternating) (p. 117)	40 sec.	2		
	Hip Bridge to Crab Rotations (p. 118)	40 sec.	2		
	Flutter Kicks with Arms over Shoulders (p. 119)	40 sec.	2		

Week 3 At-A-Glance

This week you'll do the moves EMOM-style (every minute on the minute). Begin each exercise at the start of a minute. Perform 2 reps, then use the remaining time in the minute as your rest. Repeat for a total of 15 minutes.

	WORKOUT
MONDAY	Lower-Body Moves (p. 97)
TUESDAY	Cardio
WEDNESDAY	Upper-Body Moves (p. 98)
THURSDAY	Cardio
FRIDAY	Full-Body and Core (p. 99)
SATURDAY	Cardio
SUNDAY	Rest

Tip of the Week

TEST OUT HEAVIER WEIGHTS WITH LOWER REPS.
The upper body EMOM (every minute on the minute) workout you're doing this Wednesday is the perfect opportunity to try adding a little more weight. Because there are only two repetitions per move, you should have plenty of recovery time after you complete two reps of the six moves in a set. Consider using this rest time to try raising your weights a smidge. Leslie Leal-Gauna, one of the women in our test panel, increased her weights from 8 pounds for every other workout in this book to 12 pounds for this particular workout. That doesn't mean her weights are right for you—as we know, weight selection is subjective—but it does show you that an increase is possible. Just be sure that you're using an amount of weight, a.k.a. resistance, that challenges you enough for this to feel like a struggle. As I always say, "no struggle, no story." At the end of every workout, you should have a story to tell!

LOWER-BODY MOVES

	EXERCISE	WORK	SETS	WEIGHT	NOTES
	Alternating Swings (p. 104)	2 Reps	15 min. EMOM		
	Right Lunge Back with Dumbbell Swing Backs (p. 105)	2 Reps	15 min. EMOM		
	Right Skater to Balance Holds (p. 106)	2 Reps	15 min. EMOM		
	Rainbow Lunges (p. 107)	2 Reps	15 min. EMOM		
	Left Lunge Back with Dumbbell Swing Backs (p. 105)	2 Reps	15 min. EMOM		
	Left Skater to Balance Holds (p. 106)	2 Reps	15 min. EMOM		

UPPER-BODY MOVES

	EXERCISE	WORK	SETS	WEIGHT	NOTES
	American Swings (p. 104)	2 Reps	15 min. EMOM		
	ISO Biceps Hold at 90 Degrees with Alternating Lunge Backs (p. 109)	2 Reps	15 min. EMOM		
	Reciprocal Bent-Over Rows (a.k.a., Milk the Cow) (p. 110)	2 Reps	15 min. EMOM		
	Overhead Triceps Extensions (p. 111)	2 Reps	15 min. EMOM		
	Arnold Presses (p. 112)	2 Reps	15 min. EMOM		
	90-Degree Lateral Raises (p. 113)	2 Reps	15 min. EMOM		

FULL BODY AND CORE

	EXERCISE	WORK	SETS	WEIGHT	NOTES
	Traveling Bear Planks (p. 114)	2 Reps	15 min. EMOM		
	Alternating Renegade Rows (p. 115)	2 Reps	15 min. EMOM		
	Bird Dogs (p. 116)	2 Reps	15 min. EMOM		
	Plank to Half Pigeons (Alternating) (p. 117)	2 Reps	15 min. EMOM		
	Hip Bridge to Crab Rotations (p. 118)	2 Reps	15 min. EMOM		
	Flutter Kicks with Arms over Shoulders (p. 119)	2 Reps	15 min. EMOM		

Week 4 At-A-Glance

This week you'll do the moves AMRAP-style (as many rounds as possible). Do 4 reps of each exercise with 10 seconds of rest after completing all moves. Repeat for as many rounds as possible in 20 minutes.

	WORKOUT
MONDAY	Lower-Body Moves (p.101)
TUESDAY	Cardio
WEDNESDAY	Upper-Body Moves (p. 102)
THURSDAY	Cardio
FRIDAY	Full-Body and Core (p. 103)
SATURDAY	Cardio
SUNDAY	Rest

Tip of the Week

JOURNAL YOUR SUCCESS
This week brings us to the end of this book. The first thing you should do after you complete the program is take time to appreciate how far you've come. Write down what you've learned and how you've grown along the way. Life will throw curveballs. But nothing will inspire you more than your own success story. Jot it down in your notes—on your phone or somewhere you'll always have it—so future you can find motivation in what you've accomplished over the past 28 days.

The journey doesn't stop here. As Winston Churchill said, "Now is not the end. It is not even the beginning of the end. But it is, perhaps, the end of the beginning." Pat yourself on the back for making it to the end of this beginning and know you have the knowledge—and strength!—it takes to sustain a Lift Light, Get Lean lifestyle well after you close this book.

LOWER-BODY MOVES

	EXERCISE	WORK	SETS	WEIGHT	NOTES
	Alternating Swings (p. 104)	4 Reps	20 min. AMRAP		
	Right Lunge Back with Dumbbell Swing Backs (p. 105)	4 Reps	20 min. AMRAP		
	Right Skater to Balance Holds (p. 106)	4 Reps	20 min. AMRAP		
	Rainbow Lunges (p. 107)	4 Reps	20 min. AMRAP		
	Left Lunge Back with Dumbbell Swing Backs (p. 105)	4 Reps	20 min. AMRAP		
	Left Skater to Balance Holds (p. 106)	4 Reps	20 min. AMRAP		

UPPER-BODY MOVES

	EXERCISE	WORK	SETS	WEIGHT	NOTES
	American Swings (p. 104)	4 Reps	20 min. AMRAP		
	ISO Biceps Hold at 90 Degrees with Alternating Lunge Backs (p. 109)	4 Reps	20 min. AMRAP		
	Reciprocal Bent-Over Rows (a.k.a., Milk the Cow) (p. 110)	4 Reps	20 min. AMRAP		
	Overhead Triceps Extensions (p. 111)	4 Reps	20 min. AMRAP		
	Arnold Presses (p. 112)	4 Reps	20 min. AMRAP		
	90-Degree Lateral Raises (p. 113)	4 Reps	20 min. AMRAP		

FULL BODY AND CORE

	EXERCISE	WORK	SETS	WEIGHT	NOTES
	Traveling Bear Planks (p. 114)	4 Reps	20 min. AMRAP		
	Alternating Renegade Rows (p. 115)	4 Reps	20 min. AMRAP		
	Bird Dogs (p. 116)	4 Reps	20 min. AMRAP		
	Plank to Half Pigeons (Alternating) (p. 117)	4 Reps	20 min. AMRAP		
	Hip Bridge to Crab Rotations (p. 118)	4 Reps	20 min. AMRAP		
	Flutter Kicks with Arms over Shoulders (p. 119)	4 Reps	20 min. AMRAP		

LOWER-BODY MOVES

ALTERNATING SWINGS

WHAT IT WORKS

Glutes, hamstrings, lower back, heart, and lungs

HOW TO DO IT

SETUP Holding a dumbbell in one hand, stand erect with your shoulders over your hips and legs slightly wider than hip-width apart, toes facing forward. Position the dumbbell between your thighs.

STEP 1 Hinge at the hips, driving the dumbbell between your legs up to the tops of your inner thighs.

STEP 2 Powerfully push your hips forward, propelling the weight in an arc to shoulder height. At the top of the swing, grab the weight with your other hand. Let the weight arc back to the starting position. Repeat the movement with this hand. That's 1 rep.

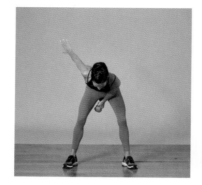
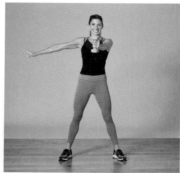
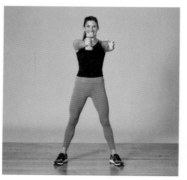
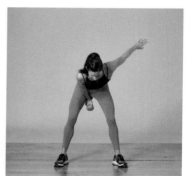

LUNGE BACK WITH A SWING BACK

WHAT IT WORKS

Quadriceps, glutes, core, and balance

HOW TO DO IT

SETUP Stand erect with your body weight primarily on your left leg with your right leg lightly propped next to it, like a kick-stand. Hold a dumbbell in your right hand. Bend your elbow to rack the dumbbell so that it is level with your right collarbone. Cup your left hand over the top of the dumbbell.

STEP 1 Lunge your right leg back, and push the dumbbell down with your left hand to accelerate a backward flow of the dumbbell to shoot it just beyond your hip.

STEP 2 Step your right leg in and bend your elbow to return the dumbbell to starting position. That's 1 rep.

NOTE

Make sure to switch your arms and legs to do the right side.

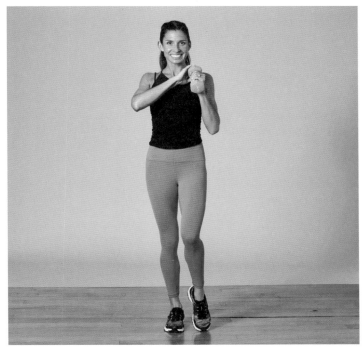

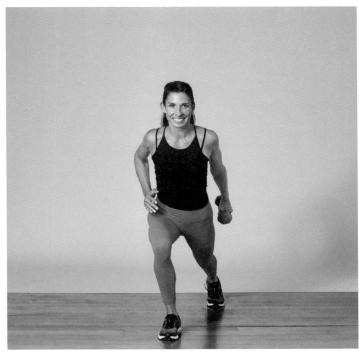

SKATER TO BALANCE HOLDS

WHAT IT WORKS

Quadriceps, sides of the glutes, hips, core, balance, heart, and lungs

HOW TO DO IT

SETUP Stand erect and balance on your right foot with your left knee and foot lifted. Bend your elbow and rack one dumbbell at your right collarbone.

STEP 1 Jump to the left side and land on your left foot with your right leg suspended behind, like a speed skater. Reach the dumbbell outside of your left knee upon landing.

STEP 2 Leap back to the right and land on your right foot with left knee lifted in starting position. That's 1 rep.

NOTE:

Make sure to switch your arms and legs to do the right side.

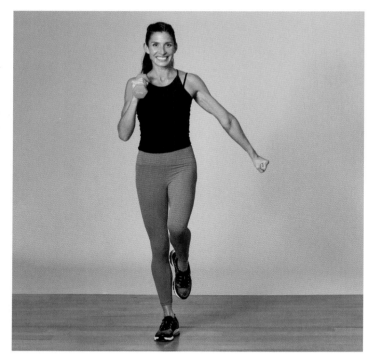

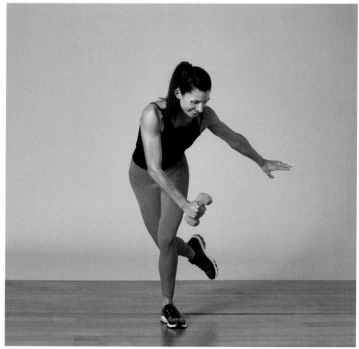

RAINBOW LUNGES

WHAT IT WORKS

Quadriceps, glutes, calves, core, shoulders, balance, heart, and lungs

HOW TO DO IT

SETUP Holding a dumbbell with both hands, stand erect with body weight evenly distributed on both feet.

STEP 1 Turn to one side and descend into a deep lunge. Hold the dumbbell between your hands in front of the lead knee.

STEP 2 Begin rising up on your legs while lifting your arms up, drawing a rainbow to the other side. Lift your heels and pivot on the balls of your feet to avoid twisting your ankles.

STEP 3 Land on the other side with the opposite knee in front and repeat the motion. That's 1 rep.

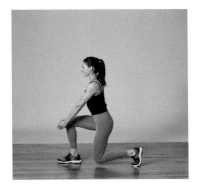
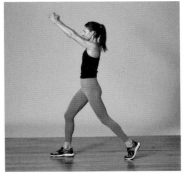
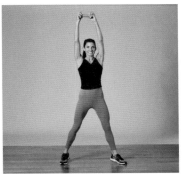
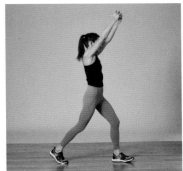
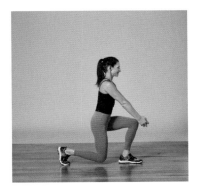

UPPER-BODY MOVES

AMERICAN SWINGS

WHAT IT WORKS

Glutes, hamstrings, lower back, shoulders, mid-back posture muscles, heart, and lungs

HOW TO DO IT

SETUP Hold a dumbbell in each hand. Stand erect with your shoulders over your hips and your legs slightly more than hip-width apart, toes facing forward.

STEP 1 Hinge at your hips, driving the dumbbells between your legs up to the tops of your inner thighs.

STEP 2 Powerfully push your hips forward, propelling the weights out until they have traveled upward in a semicircle and end up straight overhead, directly above your ears: resume your tall posture. Hold momentarily, then arc the dumbbells back to the starting position. That's 1 rep.

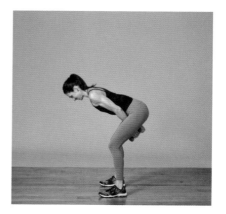

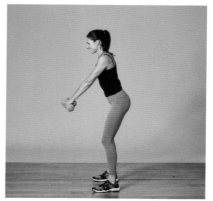

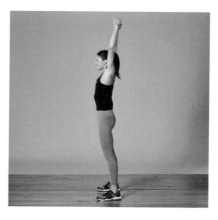

ISO BICEPS HOLD AT 90 DEGREES WITH ALTERNATING LUNGE BACK

WHAT IT WORKS

Biceps, core, quadriceps, glutes, heart, and lungs

HOW TO DO IT

SETUP Stand erect with a dumbbell in each hand, elbows glued to your sides and bent 90 degrees, forearms facing up.

STEP 1 Step one foot back into a lunge.

STEP 2 Push through your front foot and lift yourself up to starting position. Repeat on the opposite leg. That's 1 rep.

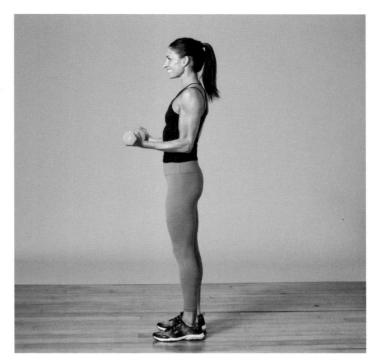

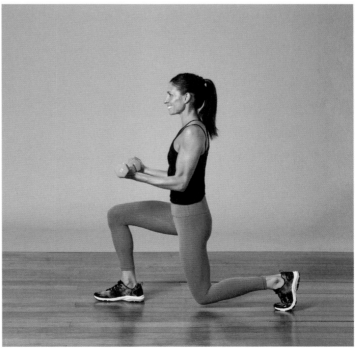

RECIPROCAL BENT-OVER ROWS (A.K.A., MILK THE COW)

WHAT IT WORKS

Back

HOW TO DO IT

SETUP Hold a dumbbell in each hand. Engage your core and tip forward at your hips, maintaining a flat back. Let your arms dangle.

STEP 1 Pull your right arm up to bring the dumbbell to your ribcage.

STEP 2 Begin slowly returning the weight to the starting position, while starting to pull your left arm to your ribcage. Both arms should hit the halfway point at the same time. When your right arm is back at the starting position, your left arm should be at your ribcage. That's 1 rep.

NOTE:

This is reciprocal, meaning both arms are moving at the same time, just in opposite directions. Your right arm is all the way up when left is all the way down and vice versa; they meet in the middle each rep.

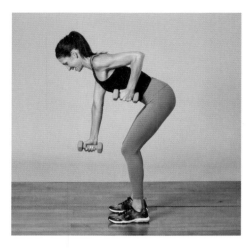
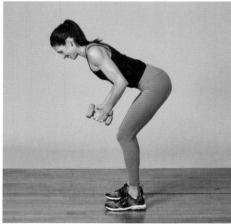
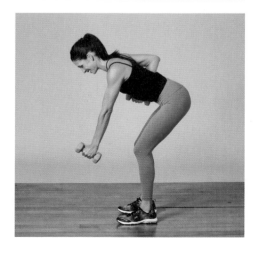

OVERHEAD TRICEPS EXTENSIONS

WHAT IT WORKS

Triceps and shoulders

HOW TO DO IT

SETUP Stand erect with a dumbbell in each hand and feet hip-width apart. Extend both arms fully overhead.

STEP 1 Keep your arms close to your head. Bend your elbows and lower the dumbbells behind your head until the dumbbells touch (or nearly touch) your shoulders. Keep your elbows pointing forward; don't let them move out to the sides.

STEP 2 Extend both elbows to return the dumbbells overhead. That's 1 rep.

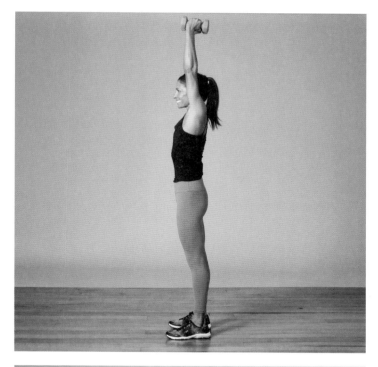

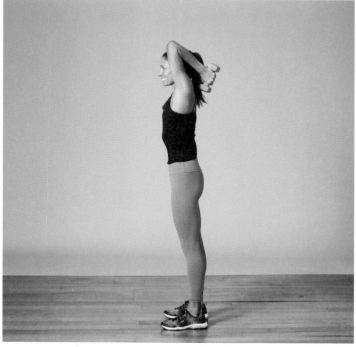

ARNOLD PRESSES

WHAT IT WORKS

Shoulders

HOW TO DO IT

SETUP Stand erect with a dumbbell in each hand. Root your feet into the floor, hip-width apart. Hold your arms with your elbows at shoulder height, forearms positioned in front of your face with palms turned in.

STEP 1 Pivot your arms out and up to push the weights straight overhead, palms facing out, with your wrists, elbows, and shoulders aligned.

STEP 2 Reverse the move to return to the starting position. That's 1 rep.

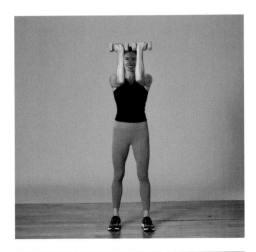

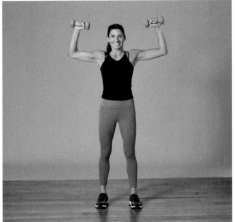

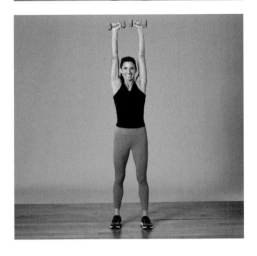

90-DEGREE LATERAL RAISES

WHAT IT WORKS

Sides of the shoulders

HOW TO DO IT

SETUP Stand erect with a dumbbell in each hand, feet hip-width apart. Root your feet into the floor. Bend your elbows to 90 degrees at your sides with elbows touching your ribcage.

STEP 1 Lift your elbows out to the sides, like you're pouring pitchers. Hold momentarily.

STEP 2 Slowly return your elbows to the starting position. That's 1 rep.

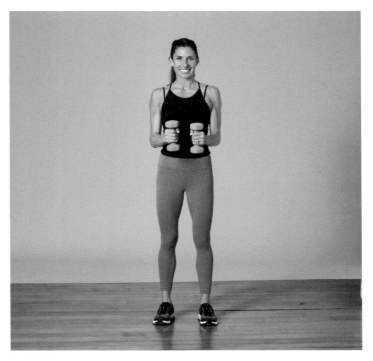

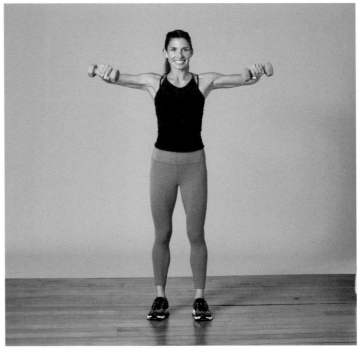

FULL BODY AND CORE

TRAVELING BEAR PLANKS

WHAT IT WORKS

Abs, shoulders, quadriceps, and glutes

HOW TO DO IT

SETUP Hold dumbbells in your hands and get into the quadruped position. Hover your knees about 1 inch above the floor.

STEP 1 Moving your right leg first, walk your feet backward to plank position, with your legs extended and your body forming a straight line from shoulders to hips to heels.

STEP 2 Starting again with your right leg, walk your feet back to the starting position. That's 1 rep.

STEP 3 Alternate lead legs every rep.

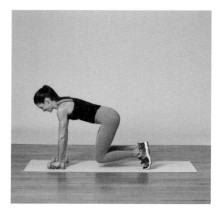

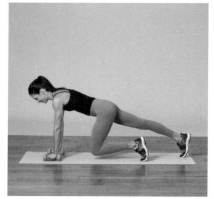

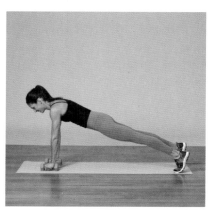

ALTERNATING RENEGADE ROWS

WHAT IT WORKS

Abs, shoulders, and back

HOW TO DO IT

SETUP Hold dumbbells in your hands underneath your shoulders and get into plank position with legs slightly more than hip-width apart—the wider your legs, the more stable you'll feel.

STEP 1 Without shifting your hips, lift one dumbbell and draw it in to touch the side of your ribcage.

STEP 2 Slowly return the weight to the floor, returning to starting position. Repeat on opposite side. That's 1 rep.

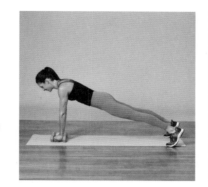
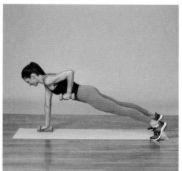

MODIFY IT!

If plank position is too challenging, use the quadruped position.

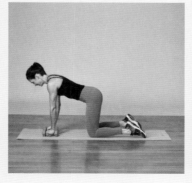
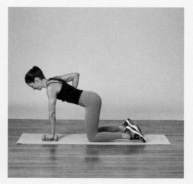

BIRD DOGS

WHAT IT WORKS

Lower back, shoulders, glutes, balance, and posture

HOW TO DO IT

SETUP Hold dumbbells in your hands and get into the quadruped position.

STEP 1 Reach one arm forward (with weight in hand) and extend the opposite leg behind you. Align both to match torso height. Hold momentarily.

STEP 2 Slowly return the arm and knee to the floor, assuming the starting position. Repeat on the opposite side. That's 1 rep.

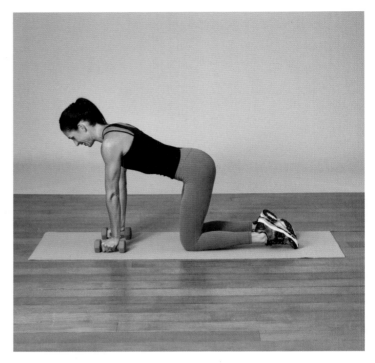

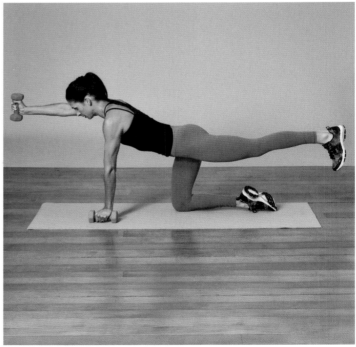

PLANK TO HALF PIGEONS (ALTERNATING)

WHAT IT WORKS

Abs, shoulders, hips, and glutes

HOW TO DO IT

SETUP Hold a dumbbell in each hand and get into plank position, hands beneath shoulders, feet about hip-width apart. There should be a straight line from shoulder to hip to heel.

STEP 1 Lift your right foot and slide that knee between your hands so your right shin is on the floor. Get into half pigeon pose: Walk your right foot toward your left hand, then lower your right thigh so it's resting on the floor, allowing your left leg to rest on the floor as well. Pull your shoulders back and open your chest wide. Hold for 1 count.

STEP 2 Grip the floor with your back toes, lift your hips to raise your right knee off the floor, and extend it back to starting position. Repeat on the opposite side. That's 1 rep.

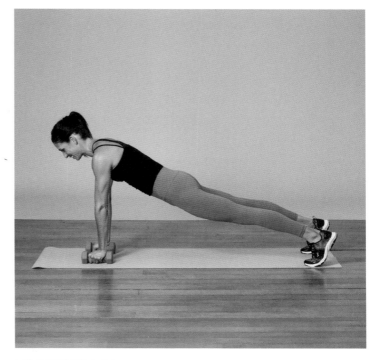

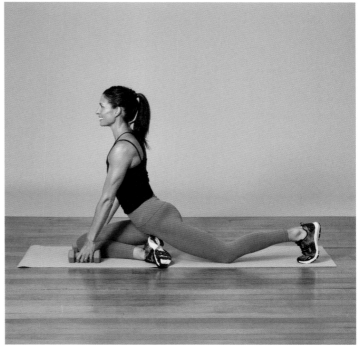

HIP BRIDGE TO CRAB ROTATIONS

WHAT IT WORKS

Shoulders, triceps, glutes, obliques, and balance

HOW TO DO IT

SETUP Hold dumbbells in your hands to keep your wrists straight and get into crab position with your butt, feet, and hands (holding the weights) on the floor, knees bent.

STEP 1 Lift your hips to form a tabletop.

STEP 2 Lower your hips to hover above the floor. Lift one leg, then lift the opposite hand and bring the weight to the outside of your lifted leg. Return to starting position.

STEP 3 Repeat with the other leg and hand. That's 1 rep.

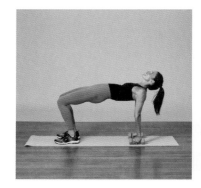
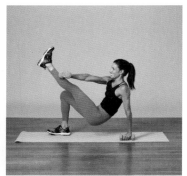
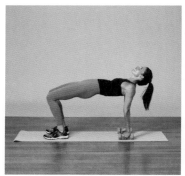
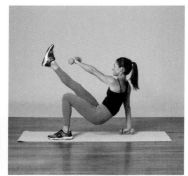

MODIFY IT!

If hovering is too difficult, keep your butt on the floor for the whole exercise.

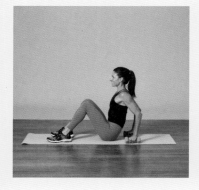
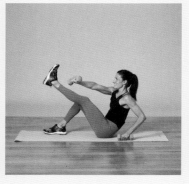

FLUTTER KICKS WITH ARMS OVER SHOULDERS

WHAT IT WORKS

Shoulders, abs, and quadriceps

HOW TO DO IT

SETUP Lie on your back and hold dumbbells straight over your shoulders. Lift your legs so they're hovering above the floor. Flex your feet. Rest your head on the floor.

STEP 1 Keeping your feet flexed, toggle the right foot above the left.

STEP 2 Keeping your feet flexed, toggle the left foot above the right. That's 1 rep.

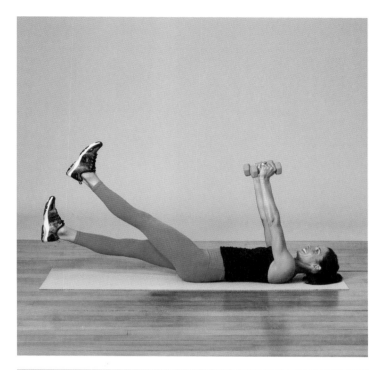

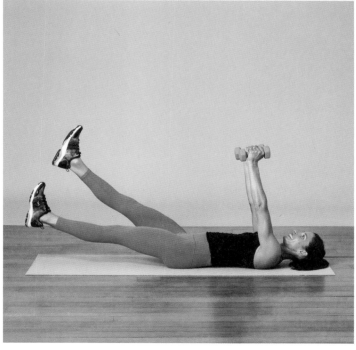

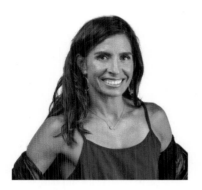

ABOUT THE AUTHOR:

Brook Benten, M.Ed., is an American College of Sports Medicine (ACSM) exercise physiologist in Austin, TX. While serving as fitness director at Southern Methodist University in Dallas, she met our nutrition contributor, Nicole Schultz. Brook was formerly a spokesperson and model for an international at-home fitness equipment company before leaving her on-camera career to serve in hospitality as Executive Director of Healthy Living at The Village Dallas. She resigned during the 2020 pandemic to be a fully present mom (pronounced "MOM!!!!!") to her two young children. Brook possesses a B.S. in Exercise and Sport Science from Texas State University (2003) and M.Ed. in Physical Education with emphasis in Sport and Fitness Administration from the University of Houston (2004). She currently writes and produces workout videos for *Prevention* Magazine.

brookbenten.com

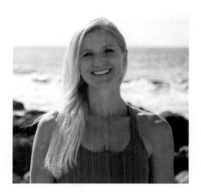

ABOUT THE CONTRIBUTORS:

Dr. Ayla Donlin, Ed.D., is a fitness and wellness professional with over 15 years of experience helping clients achieve their goals. Ayla is a certified personal trainer, wellness coach, and fitness nutrition specialist and owns a wellness coaching and consulting business, Ayla Donlin Wellness. As a mother of two girls, Ayla is passionate about empowering women to achieve their wellness goals through leveraging their strengths, exercising self-compassion, and setting priority-based boundaries.

ayladonlinwellness.com

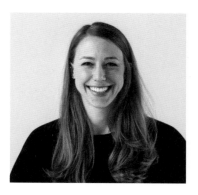

Nicole Schultz-Ninteau, Ph.D., M.P.H., C.P.T., embodies a rare combination of basic science and applied skills. Studying Human Biochemistry and Metabolism for over 12 years, Nicole simultaneously coached clients in fitness settings and taught students in academic settings. She received her bachelor's degree in Biochemistry from Southern Methodist University, and her MPH (Health Communication) and PhD (Biochemical and Molecular Nutrition with Exercise Physiology emphasis) at Tufts University. As an adjunct professor and cofounder of Enriched, she leverages her deep scientific knowledge and communication skills to elevate students' learning while leading clients to weight loss and improved eating habits.

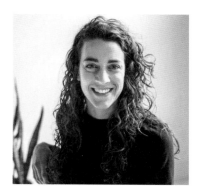

Anna Cataldo, M.S., M.P.H., R.D., Ph.D., has studied and worked in the nutrition and fitness fields for 15+ years. Her fascination with human metabolism and performance led her down a rigorous academic and clinical training path in biochemistry, exercise physiology, and nutrition science. She graduated with honors from the University of Connecticut where she studied both Exercise Physiology and Nutrition Science, received her masters degrees in Public Health and Biochemical and Molecular Nutrition from Tufts University, completed her dietetic clinical internship at Brigham and Women's Hospital and Harvard Medical School, and completed her doctorate in Rehabilitation Science at Boston University. Anna's goal is to share her knowledge and experiences in a way that helps others build confidence in and a sense of calm control over their health and well-being.

Fed up with the constant bombardment of confusing headlines and misleading nutrition information, **Nicole and Anna** founded **Enriched LLC**, an education-based company that aims to minimize the confusion around nutrition science in order to help people maximize their health and quality of life. Rather than adding to the noise, Enriched helps people navigate the nonsense and non-science surrounding nutrition by arming them with the knowledge and practical skills needed to sift through the junk. At Enriched, we translate complex scientific evidence into digestible lessons through our nutrition crash courses, consulting services, and one-on-one coaching.

enriched.health.com

NOTES

© 2023 by Hearst Magazines, Inc.

Book design by Olivia Alchek and Gillian MacLeod

Library of Congress Cataloging-in-Publication Data is on file with the publisher.

ISBN 978-1-955710-17-6

Printed in China

2 4 6 8 10 9 7 5 3 1 hardcover

HEARST

PHOTO CREDITS

Jennifer Bakos Photography: **121** (Anna Cataldo and Nicole Ninteau headshots)

Tim Dunnahoo Photography: **7, 8–9, 44, 46** (Brook Benten)

Deniz Durmas: **120** (Ayla Donlin headshot)

Philip Friedman: **Front and back cover, 5, 30–35, 55–87, 91–121, 125)**

GETTY IMAGES: Cris Cantón/Moment: **23** (water); Dave & Les Jacobs/DigitalVision: **20**; Erik Isakson/Tetra images: **48**; fcafotodigital/E+: **22** (bread); filadendron/E+: **36**; Halfpoint Images/Moment: **41**; Hinterhaus Productions/Digital Vision: **25**; JGI/Tom Grill/Tetra images: **29**; Johner Images: **23** (yogurt); kali9/E+: **27, 46, 50**; LaylaBird/E+: **18**; Nancy R. Cohen/DigitalVision: **10**; Oscar Wong/Moment: **14**; Paquito Pagulayan/EyeEm: **22** (broccoli); RunPhoto/The Image Bank: **43**; shapecharge/E+: **26**; Stanton j Stephens/Image Source: **24**; Steve Terrill/Corbis Documentary: **22** (apples); Tom Merton/OJO Images: **13, 86**; Valentyn Semenov/EyeEm: 22 (fish); Westend61: **21, 23** (avocado), **28, 42**; yacobchuk/iStock/Getty Images Plus: **17**

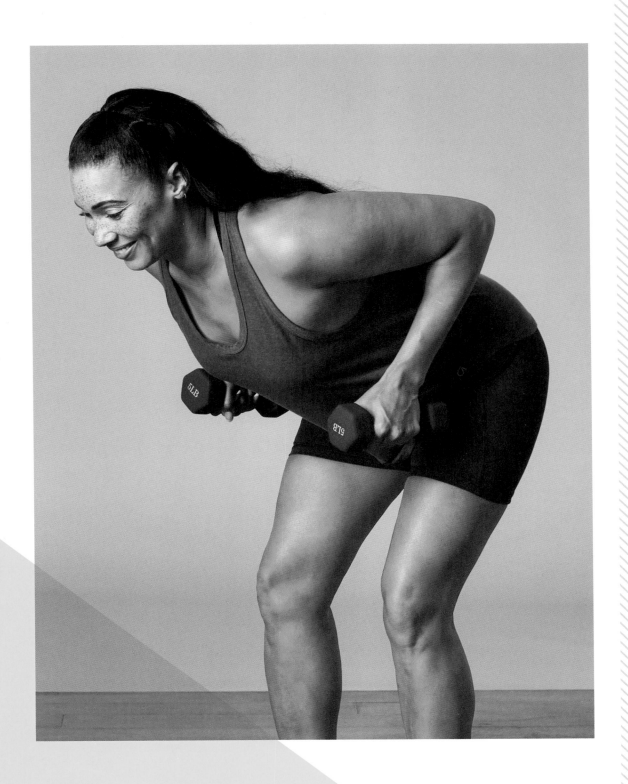

THANK YOU!

For purchasing Lift Light, Get Lean

Visit our online store to find more great products from
Prevention and save 20% off your next purchase.

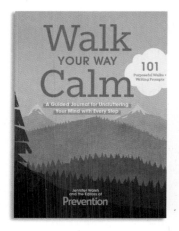
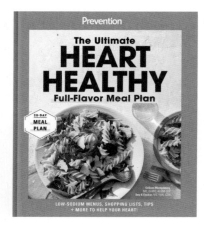
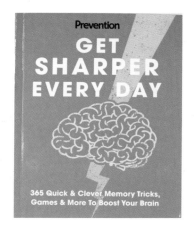

Your feedback is important to us! Scan the
QR to leave a review for Lift Light, Get Lean.

shop.prevention.com

*Exclusions Apply

HEARST